THE CARNIVORE RESET

The Primal Approach to Restoring Your Gut Health,
Reducing Inflammation, and Losing Weight

Table of Contents

Preface

I first heard about the carnivore diet back in 2016. As I'll discuss at length in this book, I was incredibly skeptical from day 1. It wasn't because I was afraid of meat either. At this point, I was almost 2 years into ketogenic diet research and had just finished my master's degree where I had the opportunity to assist with research on keto in athletes and animal models of chronic disease. I had already experienced my awakening that the mainstream narrative around red meat and fat was bogus. If you're not there yet, don't worry. This book will help with that part of your journey as well.

The reason for my skepticism came from the idea that eating only red meat would cause nutrient deficiencies. Afterall, fruits and vegetables are loaded with beneficial nutrients, right? Stay tuned. I was also skeptical because why in the world would you even need to cut out all plants? Of course, I was down with the idea of reducing carbohydrate rich foods for various health reasons but what benefit would cutting out cruciferous vegetables, low sugar fruits, and nuts and seeds provide?

The scientist in me decided that I had to give the diet a try myself and I ended up loving the way it made me feel. I had more energy, I was getting stronger and leaner, and I noticed I had a lot less joint pain that had previously plagued me from my days of playing college basketball. The results were impressive and it made me realize that like keto, carnivore could be a tool for improving body composition, energy, and athletic performance. But I didn't think the diet had much else to offer outside of that.

At the end of 2016, I heard Dr. Jordan Peterson talk about carnivore on the Joe Rogan Experience podcast. Jordan mentioned both him and his daughter Mikhaila's experience with the carnivore diet highlighting how it helped put autoimmune symptoms in remission, improved mental health, and generally led to a much better quality of life. We'll talk more about their story throughout the book. At the time, I didn't have the nutrition or biochemistry framework to help me understand how and why a carnivore diet could provide these benefits.

That podcast episode sparked a bit of a buzz in the air about this carnivore diet which led to more people trying the diet and more stories similar to the Peterson families coming out. This is when I really started to become interested in the diet.

I spent the next few years gaining a better understanding of autoimmune conditions, gut health, and the many compounds found in plants that could impact these areas of health. Combined with a growing number of anecdotal stories, it was becoming obvious that carnivore was a lot more than just a ancestral way of eating to lose weight. The diet clearly had potential for therapeutic use.

Over the last couple of years, the carnivore diet has continued to gain traction which, like any diet, has led to this way of eating being labeled a "fad". This has in part been due to the growing number of extreme carnivore personas, like Liver King, who have been born out of this booming ancestral lifestyle. The carnivore diet has also been put through the ringer being labeled a "right wing" way of eating that fails to take into account the health of our environment and the rights of animals.

Combined with a society wide fear of red meat, a perfect storm has been created, leading to carnivore becoming something that it is not and many forgetting what the diet really can be. Thousand of people have found incredible healing from autoimmune conditions, mental health disorders, and both extreme and minor digestive complications. If this is a fad diet, then I think we need to reconsider the therapeutic utilization of fad diets.

The reason I set out to write the Carnivore Reset is to both remind people of the therapeutic potential of carnivore and to help the growing number of people who are dealing with autoimmune disease and poor gut health who have been failed by our conventional healthcare system. As you read this book, my goal is to help drown out the noise from health "experts" telling you that its all about calories, that meat is bad for your health and the environment, and that carnivore is a fad diet with no therapeutic potential. The science and the anecdotal evidence is there and in this book we are going to present all of it to you.

Enjoy,

Chris Irvin "The Ketologist"

Introduction

Whether she knew it or not, Megan had suffered from poor digestive health since she was a teenager. In high school, she recalls her "embarrassingly horrific acne," which she could never get under control no matter how many topical steroidal medications she tried.

In Megan's early years of college, she encountered a new, seemingly separate problem when she developed a gluten intolerance. While it wasn't the crippling digestive pain that some people experience, it made for an unpleasant morning after a night of eating pizza (and enjoying a few beers) with her friends.

After college, Megan found that she continued to develop different food intolerances. First, it was dairy, then eggs began to bother her, and eventually, even certain vegetables would put her stomach in a bind. While she didn't make the connection at the time, her anxiety, which was always present in the background during her younger years, started taking center stage in her life. While her digestive issues were taking a toll on her body, her anxiety affected her professional life and personal relationships, leaving her feeling like a shell of herself.

Before Megan came to Chris for help, she had reached a point where her digestive system was almost always giving her trouble. Simple activities like going out to eat, enjoying appetizers at a party, or even taking care of her day-to-day activities turned into moments of pain, discomfort, and, in some cases, experiences of intense embarrassment.

Does this sound familiar? If not as severe, maybe to a lesser extent? If not you, maybe someone you know?

Roughly 11% of the US population suffers from chronic digestive diseases[1]. That's over 36 million people and doesn't account for the minor, more common digestive issues like bloating, stomach pain, constipation, and diarrhea that affect nearly two-thirds of the US population[2]. Given that you're reading this right now, we'll assume you may have a place somewhere in those statistics, and we can assure you that no matter what physicians have told you, feeling uncomfortable every time you eat is not normal. But it is fixable.

Maybe you've been dealing with digestive problems for a while and have tried just about everything. You've gone gluten-free, dairy-free, low FODMAP, and, of course, you've tried every supplement under the sun. While your intentions have been good, at the end of the day, it seems like the more time and money you spend, the worse your symptoms get.

Or, perhaps you're doing fine; you don't have any extreme symptoms (yet), but you frequently feel bloated after eating or experience discomfort after consuming certain foods, and a coworker told you that it might be your gut health so you did a google search and found this book.

Or, maybe you aren't experiencing any digestive issues but are struggling with weight loss, hormone balance, mood, or inflammation. The truth is that your digestive system plays a major role in nearly every aspect of your health, and a healthy gut is a key player in achieving any health goal and just better overall wellness.

It should come as no surprise that when dealing with gut health, what you eat matters, and in some instances, there's just no supplement or drug that can solve the problem.

Your gut might be damaged, and you don't even know it. Like Megan, you might be suffering from acne, brain fog, or joint pain, which seemingly has nothing to do with the gut. But gut issues can disguise themselves as all sorts of unusual problems that are often treated with bandaids. Instead of trying to cover up your symptoms, which we'll admit can be tempting, we want to help you get to the root of it.

Whatever your motivation may be, the Carnivore Reset was created not only to educate you on gut health but to offer a potential solution with the ultimate elimination diet - the carnivore diet.

Why Carnivore?

We know what you're thinking; "Isn't meat causing all the problems - destroying our health and the environment as we speak!? How could it possibly be that we've gone from fruits and vegetables being all the rage to now…meat?"

This may take some time to wrap your head around, and we'll spend ample time explaining it, but the truth is that meat is not the problem. Even more surprising is that plants may actually be the source of your problems.

The problem is that we value plant-based foods so highly that we create a blind spot, convincing ourselves that there's no way these foods could possibly be the issue. How could vegetables, with all of their nutrients and fiber, possibly steer us wrong?

Amazingly, what we've found time and again is that when we help people remove plants from their diet, they find relief from their bloating and other digestive discomforts. And for most of these people, it doesn't take long to start feeling the effects. In many cases, people feel relief immediately.

The reason for this is both complex and straightforward: we need modern solutions to modern problems.

Now, some would say that this isn't a modern solution because humans have a long history of carnivorous eating. This is true. But even among the most carnivore of our ancestors, complete avoidance of plant foods was not really a thing. Our hunter-gatherer ancestors often consumed edible plants when the opportunity presented itself; they just didn't eat very much because these opportunities were often scarce.

Why wouldn't they? Hundreds of years ago, when people were consuming most of their food off the land and in a package that nature intended (i.e., whole and unprocessed), it's unlikely that anyone would have needed to take such drastic measures as the complete removal of plants from their diet to find digestive relief. It's also unlikely that our ancestors suffered from the kind of digestive discomfort that we see today.

Unfortunately, our diets today are far from what our ancestors ate. Even as little as a hundred years ago, we would see considerably fewer processed foods on the shelves of grocery stores. Due to the nature of our modern food system, our digestion has been put to the test with excess sugar, artificial ingredients, preservatives, and plant compounds that would likely have been removed in a more natural cooking process or consumed in much smaller quantities.

Are plants 100% to blame for our digestive issues? Likely not. In fact, it would be remiss for us not to mention the impact that emotional stress can have on gut health, which is an epidemic all its own these days. And, of course, toxins, additives, and artificial ingredients in our foods have only added to the problem.

While plants may not always be the cause or the only triggering factor, they are certainly a factor that can propagate gut issues and prevent healing. This is the information that most well-intentioned people are missing when they try to eliminate "triggering" foods while consuming a diet rich in plant foods.

All of this to say, don't get the wrong idea; the information in this book is not meant to scare you away from plants. We don't believe completely eliminating plants from your diet for the rest of your life is necessarily the way to go (unless you are dealing with more severe cases of chronic autoimmunity). Instead, we want to educate you on both plant and animal foods to help you identify which foods and in what quantities your body has difficulty tolerating.

In the last few years, the carnivore diet has been popularized by people like Mikhaila Peterson (now Mikhaila Fuller), Dr. Paul Saladino, and Dr. Shawn Baker - the leaders of the carnivore movement, so to speak. The growth of this movement, with hundreds of thousands of people adopting this style of eating, has shed light on the powers of the carnivore diet. While we love rigorous scientific evidence as much as the next person, which the carnivore diet currently lacks, there are just too many anecdotes that we simply can't ignore anymore (hence the creation of this book).

People are reversing autoimmune disorders, effortlessly losing weight, curing digestive issues, and ultimately regaining their health by eliminating plants from their diet. We've also both experimented with the diet several times ourselves, with Cynthia taking the (steak) cake with her personal story.

In 2019, Cynthia was hospitalized for 13 days due to a ruptured appendix that came with a plethora of complications, including a small bowel obstruction, pancolitis, retroperitoneal abscesses, and a fistula. During her hospitalization, she received antibiotics, antifungal agents, TPN, and total parenteral nutrition, which is nutrition in intravenous form. She underwent multiple procedures, including special drains to help her fistula drain and having a peripheral IV line put in. Interestingly, during the course of her hospitalization, she intensely craved salt, water, AND meat. She even dreamt of "juicy burgers."

After her hospitalization and, ultimately, an appendectomy, she experienced 6+ months of debilitating diarrhea, which led the healthcare team to recommend a "low residue" diet. Most foods on a low-residue diet are typically devoid of any nutritional value and are highly processed. Interestingly, Cynthia noticed that the only thing that didn't upset her stomach during this time was braised/gently cooked meat. She craved salt and loved bone broth and stew meats.

All of this led to Cynthia deciding to give this carnivore diet a shot. Thankfully, her gastroenterologist and surgeon were very supportive, and the response was incredible. Shortly after starting the diet, Cynthia saw a normalization of gut motility, less bloating/cramping, less inflammation, and just a feeling of better overall digestion. Eventually, Cynthia did start to miss vegetables and decided to work to incorporate them back into her diet as tolerated (we'll get to that in the reintroduction phase) but noticed that she had a new sensitivity to oxalates, which helped her understand which vegetables to stay away from. In this book, we'll help you figure out the same.

Together, we created this book as a tool to give you a step-by-step process outlining what you need to give your gut the reset it deserves so you can finally experience how food should make you feel.

We want to preface the rest of this book by saying that science has yet to provide us with the long-term effects of a carnivore diet. With this in mind, we aren't advising you to follow a strict carnivore diet for life (although some cases may require this). Instead, the purpose of this writing is to promote gut rest by eliminating the most common dietary triggers of digestive upset, thus allowing you the opportunity to learn about your body and experience what it feels like to live without digestive discomfort. Once you've gained control over your symptoms, you'll be able to design the optimal diet for your unique body so you can feel your best and thrive going forward.

In this book, you'll find a protocol that allows you to achieve just that. The elimination phase of that protocol is followed by the opportunity to identify individual food intolerances through a reintroduction phase. Everyone is different, and the gut is a unique and mysterious place that scientists are still trying to understand. You might come to learn that you do well with certain plants while others leave you feeling horrible. For some people, eating a carnivore or mostly carnivore diet is going to be the best strategy for the long haul, and others may find after this program that they can "tolerate" all plants again. Your experience will be unique to you, but let's just say you're in for an eye-opening experience.

Disclaimer: The information here is not medical advice and is not to be misconstrued as a medical treatment.

Alright, let's jump in.

Chapter 1:

Gut Health 101

"All Disease Begins in The Gut." - Hippocrates.

The quote above dates back nearly 2,500 years ago. Did Hippocrates have it right all along?

Mainstream medicine will often overlook the role the gut plays in our overall health, and it's certainly not common for gut health to be considered the root of any health issues. But the truth is that your gut plays such an essential role in your health that not considering its impact is ludicrous.

Many health issues are influenced by what we eat, dictated at large by the current state of our metabolic health and the status of our gut. Unless you're running extensive labs on yourself, you may not even realize how your diet could be hurting you. It gets even more confusing when supposedly "healthy" foods are irritating your gut and setting you back. Why does that happen? How does food become public enemy number one? If you're feeling a little overwhelmed, don't worry – once you understand the structure and function of your gut, this will start to make a lot more sense.

Two of the major determinants of gut health are the gut barrier and the gut microbiome.

Our diet impacts both of these factors since our food comes into direct contact with both the gut barrier and the microbiome multiple times per day (for most people). If you're regularly eating something that's upsetting your gut, at some point, you're likely to experience issues due to either or both of these components of the gut becoming compromised to some degree. Your gut is only so resilient.

Let's start with the gut barrier.

The Gut Barrier and Leaky Gut

The gut barrier is the lining of the digestive tract, also known as the intestinal barrier. It's the middleman between the outside world and the inside of our bodies. What's fascinating about this incredibly important component of our gut is that it's made up of just a SINGLE layer of epithelial cells covered by a layer of mucus that adds a little extra protection.

The gut barrier has many roles:

Roles of The Gut Barrier

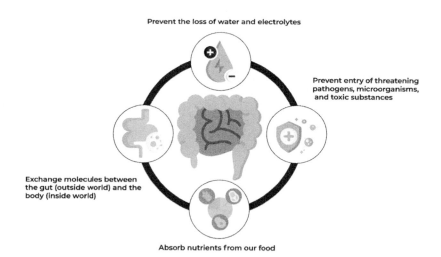

Prevent the loss of water and electrolytes

Prevent entry of threatening pathogens, microorganisms, and toxic substances

Exchange molecules between the gut (outside world) and the body (inside world)

Absorb nutrients from our food

Put simply, the gut barrier lets the good guys in while keeping the bad guys out. Or, that's its intention, at least. When all is functioning optimally, an impressive balancing act exists between uptake and exclusion from the foods we eat.

Again, just a thin layer of cells acts as the line of defense against potentially harmful substances in our food from entering our bloodstream and moving throughout our bodies. Needless to say, this layer of cells is kind of important.

While the gut barrier is capable of incredible feats, it's also very vulnerable to damage. Alas, our poor diets flooded with refined carbs, insulting vegetable oils, chemical agents, and a surplus of other compounds we probably shouldn't be consuming pose the risk of damaging the gut's sensitive lining.

Food that enters the intestine first encounters the mucus layer of the gut barrier. The mucus layer acts as the first line of physical defense, preventing pathogens from contacting the layer of intestinal epithelial cells that lay beneath. Essentially, the mucus layer is a gel-like protectant for the epithelial cells. It's not only a physical barrier but also hosts antimicrobial proteins and antibodies that chemically defend against pathogens.

Below the mucus layer, the cells of the gut lining are held together by proteins known as tight junctions. With the help of these tight junctions, the gut barrier remains selectively permeable, meaning when they are functioning optimally, they only let items pass through the barrier that are supposed to. However, if these tight junctions are damaged, they loosen up, and intestinal permeability increases, allowing foreign invaders to breach the gut barrier and enter our bloodstream.

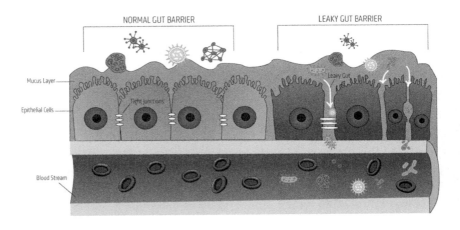

In short, intestinal permeability is the term that describes the level of control the gut barrier has over what gets through. Healthy intestinal permeability is dependent on a healthy gut microbiome (I'll get to that in a second), healthy mucus layer, and intact tight junctions.

In the mainstream, increased intestinal permeability is more commonly known as **leaky gut**. Again, a "leaky" gut means there are gaps between the cells of the gut barrier (damaged tight junctions), allowing for the entry of pathogens and toxins across the gut barrier to invade the body.

This is bad news.

When bacteria and bacterial products (e.g., lipopolysaccharides (LPS), pathogenic microorganisms, toxins, etc.) cross the gut barrier, the body tries to get rid of them by activating the immune system, which calls the troops in for battle. By troops, we mean inflammatory molecules that intend to fight off the invaders but can also drive up systemic inflammation in the process. This is essentially the body's alarm system, signaling the presence of intruders.

There's a building consensus within the scientific community that a leaky gut can be a source of chronic inflammation[1], which makes sense as to why a leaky gut has ties with several inflammatory health problems. Increased gut permeability (leaky gut) is a common denominator of autoimmune disorders[2], inflammatory bowel diseases[3], celiac disease[4], food allergies[5], irritable bowel syndrome[6], and more recently recognized in obesity and metabolic diseases[7]. Damage to the gut barrier may be due to direct damage by certain foods and food additives and/or changes in the gut microbiome that affect the barrier's integrity.

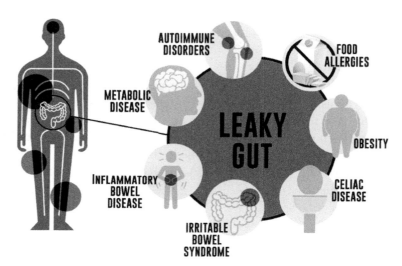

We should all be striving for optimal intestinal permeability so that the gut barrier is only permeable to the nutrients and molecules that our body needs while being impermeable to potential threats.

Gut Barrier Glossary/Summary

Intestinal Barrier: The physical barrier/gut wall separating the inside of the intestines (gut lumen) from the inside of the body (i.e., bloodstream). Its role is to let nutrients in and keep pathogens out, and also hosts a significant component of the immune system.

Intestinal Permeability: The degree of control the gut barrier has over what gets into the body and is dependent on the structure and function of the intestinal barrier.

Leaky gut: The common term to describe impaired intestinal permeability as a result of physical damage to the gut wall. This means the gut has lost control over what can pass ("leak") through into the body.

Ok, on to the gut microbiome.

Gut Microbiome

The gut microbiome is another rapidly growing area of research that triggers more questions than answers. Research on the gut microbiome is still in its infancy, and there is still an enormous amount of information left to decode.

Here's what we know so far.

Inside each and every one of us is a whole separate world hosting trillions of microorganisms that are ideally working with us in symbiosis, keeping us healthy and thriving. This world exists in our digestive tract and consists of bacteria, viruses, fungi, and other microorganisms. The most abundant bacteria in the gut microbiome are Bacteroidetes and Firmicutes, but other prevalent strains include Actinobacteria, Proteobacteria, and Verrucomicrobia.

The gut microbiome assists in processing and digesting the food we eat so that we can absorb the energy and nutrients locked inside. But it does a lot more than that. It also helps food move through the intestines, regulates blood sugar levels, synthesizes vitamins, and is in constant communication with our immune system[8,9,10]. It even communicates with the brain, affecting mood, appetite, and brain function[11,12,] and plays a significant role in regulating metabolism and energy balance. Of importance, the gut microbiome also helps maintain proper gut barrier function, so it has an important relationship with leaky gut[13].

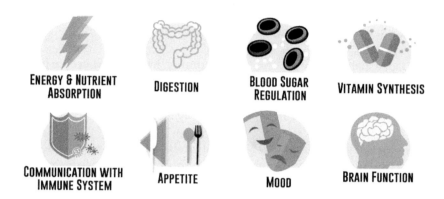

| ENERGY & NUTRIENT ABSORPTION | DIGESTION | BLOOD SUGAR REGULATION | VITAMIN SYNTHESIS |

| COMMUNICATION WITH IMMUNE SYSTEM | APPETITE | MOOD | BRAIN FUNCTION |

Dysbiosis is the term we use when the gut microbiome is out of balance or, rather when there is a decrease in beneficial gut bacteria and an increase in harmful bacteria. Dysbiosis is linked to a litany of health complications, including digestive issues like inflammatory bowel disease and even obesity, anxiety, and type 2 diabetes.

This may come as a surprise, but there's not a single blueprint for an optimal healthy gut microbiome. Cultures around the world have existed and thrived eating a wide variety of different foods, all requiring different gut microbes that support their specific diet. The gut microbiome is highly adaptable and changes rapidly (in as little as 48 hours) based on what we feed it[14].

The adaptability of the gut microbiome was likely established during evolution, in concert with our body's ability to switch between burning carbohydrates to fats and ketones depending on what, or if, food was available at any given time. If food was scarce, or if animal foods were the only thing available, the gut microbiome would shift to accommodate for this. In fact, one study compared the gut microbiomes of healthy humans following a short-term plant-based diet or animal-based diet (which was also ketogenic)[14]. The results showed that the animal-based diet caused an increase in strains that metabolize fats and a decrease in those known to metabolize carbohydrates - the type of results you would expect on an animal-based diet. This doesn't say anything about an animal-based diet promoting pathogenic bacteria or supporting a beneficial microbiome, but rather that the gut can respond appropriately to different food sources.

We see similar results in a separate study that looked at the seasonal changes to the gut microbiome of the Hadza hunter-gatherers, whose diet changes profoundly with the seasons[15].

The Hadza tribe is one of the few remaining hunter-gatherer tribes in Africa, living entirely off the land with no domesticated livestock or food storage. Hunting with hand-made bows and foraging edible plants, the Hazda exemplify the true meaning of eating seasonally.

During the dry season, from May to October, they consume plentiful amounts of meat; during the wet season, from November to April, they rely more heavily on berries. As their diets change with each season, their gut microbiome shifts accordingly.

What's interesting about tribes like the Hadza or even the Inuit, who also rely heavily on high-fat animal foods, is that their people have no apparent gut issues and are largely free of most chronic diseases.

Despite this, high-fat diets get a bad rap as far as the gut microbiome goes. Why? Shoddy science has led to the publication of several studies that seem to show the detrimental effects of "high-fat diets" when what they're really highlighting is the effects of health-damaging fats like vegetable oils, along with refined sugar and toxic plant compounds— nothing like the foods you eat on a carnivore diet.

Do you know which diets are associated with gut issues? Western diets that are high in sugar, processed vegetable oils, and refined grains[16]. These diets disrupt the gut microbiome and encourage the growth of harmful bacterial strains while starving off the good bacteria.

The Estrobolome

The gut microbiome can be further broken down into more specific subparts, such as the estrobolome. The estrobolome refers to a collection of bacteria in the gut microbiome that interact with estrogens[17].

Once estrogens have completed their circulation in the bloodstream and through our various organs/tissues, the body works diligently to properly break down estrogen for either elimination or reabsorption. This begins with estrogen molecules being sent to the liver to undergo phase 1 clearance, where estrogen is reduced down to a less active form, and phase 2, where it undergoes conjugation, becoming bonded to glucuronic acid, which makes the estrogen molecule less active and more water-soluble in preparation for elimination. Conjugated estrogens are then funneled to the kidneys or the intestinal tract to be eliminated via urine and feces in what is considered phase 3 of the elimination process.

Conjugated estrogens that make it to the intestinal tract are subject to the current state of the gut microbiome, or more specifically, the estrobolome, where they can experience one of two fates. If the estrobolome contains a low number of both deconjugating bacteria and deconjugating enzymes like beta-glucuronidase, then the conjugated estrogens are eliminated through fecal excretion. If the estrobolome has high levels of deconjugating bacteria and enzymes, the conjugated estrogens can be deconjugated and reabsorbed into the bloodstream through the intestines. All of which can potentially contribute to an imbalance in circulating estrogen levels.

Dramatically increasing or decreasing circulating estrogen levels can have a big impact on many aspects of women's health. As it relates to this book, it can further impact gut health by altering gut motility and inflammation and facilitating digestive disorders like IBS, IBD, and GERD through estrogen receptors found in the gut.

Estrobolome health can be monitored through stool analysis that looks at gut microbiota composition, urinary metabolite testing looking at different estrogen metabolites in the urine, and blood tests looking at circulating estrogen levels and even markers of liver health. There are also symptoms and side effects of poor estrobolome health worth paying attention to, like PMS, endometriosis, PCOS, breast pain, cyclical fertility challenges, uterine fibroids, and more.

Similar to the gut microbiome in general, there are many factors that influence estrobolome health, including diet and medications like antibiotics. While there is no research looking at the impact of the carnivore diet on the estrobolome specifically, given what we know about the microbiome as a whole, if the estrobolome is compromised with an overgrowth of the wrong kind of bacteria, carnivore can potentially help by starving those bacteria off and giving you a chance to reset the gut.

Lipopolysaccharides

A major component of the gut microbiome and the harm it can produce is the presence of lipopolysaccharides or LPS. LPS are large molecules synthesized by certain types of bacteria found in our gut. When LPS is created, it's transported to and embedded in the outer surface of the bacterial membrane. From here, the LPS molecule can be shed from the surface of the bacteria and enter the gut environment.

LPS are known as endotoxins because they can cause harmful effects in the body. For example, they can stimulate inflammatory cytokines to drive up gut inflammation and disrupt the balance of the gut microbiome, leading to the overgrowth of harmful bacteria. They can also cause leaky gut, which allows this compound to enter the bloodstream, where it can trigger a systemic inflammatory response. For these reasons, LPS is linked to a range of gut disorders, including IBD and IBS.

Several factors, including a high-sugar diet, alcohol consumption, stress, and bacterial infections, can all stimulate LPS.

Symptoms of Poor Gut Health

Now that you understand the importance and complexity of your gut let's talk about the symptoms and causes of poor gut health.

Poor gut health can manifest itself rather erratically, affecting areas of your health that you may never have linked to your gut. Here's a short list of the symptoms that can be experienced from poor gut health:

* Chronic constipation
* Frequent bloating
* Diarrhea
* Obesity
* Food intolerances
* Gas
* Stomach pain
* Depression
* Anxiety
* Acne
* Eczema
* Menstrual irregularities
* Psoriasis
* Autoimmune disease

Every individual with poor gut health may experience these symptoms differently. Some will only experience them occasionally, and some will experience them daily. Some may only experience one of these symptoms, while others experience several. Some people, like Megan in the introduction, may even experience different symptoms at different stages of their life.

One of the biggest problems with having poor gut health is that many of these symptoms are often not associated with gut health by mainstream healthcare. Instead, they're often chalked up to other problems and even treated as other problems. This is a big reason why many people dealing with poor gut health very rarely experience a cure or even improvements throughout their lives.

Causes of Poor Gut Health

Knowing that you have poor gut health is one thing, but trying to get to the root of it is a whole other story. Unfortunately, what makes healing your gut issues so confusing is the wide variety of potential contributors.

While it's likely that the biggest contributors are those coming from your diet, which we'll get to in a second, it's important to know that many other aspects of your lifestyle can also contribute to poor gut health. Exercise[18], sleep[19], and stress[20] all have the ability to impact your gut microbiome, setting you up for better or worse digestive health.

With that being said, we still believe that what we put in our bodies is the most significant contributor to poor gut health. Still, even within this category, there are several potential contributors. Let's go over a few:

Seed Oils

Seed oils or vegetable oils are cooking oils that are used entirely too much in our society. They include sunflower, peanut, safflower, corn, soybean, canola, cottonseed, and canola oil. You can find these oils on the ingredient list of nearly every packaged food (even the foods labeled "healthy"), and they're used as cooking oils at most restaurants (even the "healthy" restaurants).

The problem with seed oils is multifaceted. Seed oils are rich in omega-6 fatty acids. While omega-6 fats often get a bad reputation as being proinflammatory, they're actually essential to our health. We just shouldn't be consuming as much of them as we are. The recommended ratio of omega-6 to omega-3 fatty acids is somewhere between 1:1 and 4:1. This ratio is key to keeping inflammation in check. If you're following the

Standard American Diet, then you're likely eating a ratio closer to 20:1. A recipe for inflammation, and as we covered earlier in the book, inflammation is a key player in dysfunctional gut health.

Even worse, these seed oils are not stable, meaning at high temperatures, they become oxidized, allowing them to become even more pro-inflammatory. When cooking with these oils, especially frying, we're doing just that.

Refined seed oils have been linked to many adverse effects on gut health, including the disruption of bacterial balance in the microbiome. Seed oils are also highly refined and treated with chemicals to remove unpleasant taste and smell. These chemicals can be disruptive to our gut by damaging the intestinal lining and promoting a leaky gut. In one study[21], researchers found that a diet high in linoleic acid, a type of omega-6 found in refined seed oils, resulted in an increase in gut permeability, which, as you now know, can contribute to inflammation and other digestive issues.

Refined Carbs

Refined carbohydrates, which are often found in processed foods, have also been linked to negative effects on gut health. These types of carbohydrates are quickly digested and absorbed by the body, leading to rapid spikes in blood sugar levels. This can disrupt the balance of healthy bacteria in the gut, leading to an increase in harmful bacteria and a decrease in beneficial bacteria. Research published in the journal Nutrients found that a diet high in refined carbohydrates led to a decrease in the diversity of the gut microbiome[22]. Another study found that a diet high in refined carbohydrates led to an increase in inflammation in the gut[23].

Alcohol

Chronic alcohol consumption can also pose a serious problem when it comes to our gut health.

One study examined the gut microbiome of 48 alcoholics and compared them to a group of 18 healthy individuals who consumed little or no alcohol. The researchers found that 23% of the alcoholic population showed signs of dysbiosis, whereas none of the healthy individuals did[24]. Another study looking at the effects of different types of alcohol on gut bacteria found that gin led to a decrease in beneficial gut bacteria[25]. Yet another study found that consuming high levels of alcohol can lead to an increase in intestinal permeability[26].

Antibiotic Use

Antibiotic use can have a significant impact on gut health, as antibiotics can kill gut bacteria and thus disrupt the natural balance of the gut microbiome. A systematic review of antibiotic use and the microbiome found that antibiotics were associated with decreased microbial diversity and alterations in the composition of the gut microbiome[27]. In another study, researchers found that the impact of antibiotics on microbial diversity continued to persist two years later[28]!

Perhaps even more alarming is that many studies show that antibiotic use can lead to the expansion of antibiotic-resistant bacteria in the gut, which may increase the risk of infections and other health problems[29].

Cigarette Smoking

Research has found that smoking is also associated with alterations in the gut microbiome, including decreased microbial diversity and changes in the abundance of specific bacteria[30], an increase in intestinal permeability, and an increased risk of inflammatory bowel disease (IBD), including Crohn's disease and ulcerative colitis[31].

Even better is a study that found that smoking cessation increased beneficial bacteria in the gut[32], highlighting that if you are a smoker, stopping can make a big difference on your gut health!

Chronic Stress

Surprisingly, chronic stress can also disrupt gut health33. Stress hormones can alter gut motility, the movement of food through the digestive tract, leading to symptoms like constipation or diarrhea. Stress can also impact the secretion of digestive juices, potentially leading to indigestion and/ or acid reflux.

Chronic stress can compromise the integrity of the gut lining, increasing leaky gut and allowing harmful substances to enter the bloodstream, potentially triggering inflammation and immune responses. Stress can also adversely affect the gut microbiome and lead to poor dietary choices that can further exacerbate digestive problems.

Hormone Changes

Hormonal fluctuations and shifts, particularly during a woman's menstrual cycle, pregnancy, post-partum, perimenopause, and menopause, can significantly impact gut health. In fact, fluctuations in key hormones like estrogen and progesterone can influence digestive function as a whole. High levels of estrogen can speed up transit time or digestion, leading to looser stools and increased bowel movement frequency, which is not always a good thing. On the other hand, progesterone tends to slow down digestion, leading to a longer transit time, which could lead to constipation. Both can have an impact on the gut microbiome.

This is a big reason why many women experience changes in bowel habits during menstruation, including increases in digestive symptoms like bloating, constipation, or diarrhea. During pregnancy, increased progesterone can slow down digestion and cause issues like constipation and gastroesophageal reflux[34]. Postmenopause leads to decreased estrogen levels, which can affect gut function[35], potentially altering the gut microbiome and contributing to gastrointestinal conditions.

It is also worth mentioning that estrogen and progesterone can have a big impact on the immune system as well, which, as you will see throughout this book, can also influence gut health, especially in those dealing with autoimmunity.

Water Supply

Without being too much of an alarmist here, it's important to point out that even our water can impact our gut health. More specifically, tap water. Depending on where you are located, tap water can be loaded with potentially toxic compounds, including disinfection byproducts (DBPs), which are formed when water treatment compounds like chlorine combine with natural compounds found in water. One study found that exposure to DBPs in tap water resulted in alterations in the gut microbiome, explicitly targeting the microbiota and decreasing diversity[36].

Studies have also investigated the presence of microplastics in tap water and their potential impact on human health. Research shows that microplastics may lead to changes in the gut microbiome and encourage intestinal permeability[37].

In addition to DBPs and microplastics, depending on where you live, your tap water could also be contaminated with a myriad of other toxic compounds. Heavy metals, pharmaceuticals, PFAS (also known as "forever chemicals"), nitrates, and radioactive nucleotides are just a handful.

Meal Frequency

Even the frequency with which you consume food can have an impact on your gut health. Under ancestral conditions, you would only eat when food was available – which might amount to one or two times a day (maybe three if you were really fortunate). Now, it's common practice to eat more meals and snack between meals, leading to a near-constant intake of food.

The consequence of this high eating frequency is a digestive system that gets worn out. One study looking at the impact of scheduled eating breaks (AKA intermittent fasting) found that giving yourself space between meals could improve microbial diversity, specifically favoring the growth and proliferation of anti-inflammatory bacteria[38].

A systematic review examining the impact of intermittent fasting on the gut microbiome found that leaving space between meals improved the diversity and abundance of gut microbes, particularly of those species associated with metabolic health. The investigators noted that once people returned to a more frequent eating pattern, some of those changes were reversed[39].

Plant Compounds

We saved this one for last because, as surprising as it may sound, if you have tried a bunch of other diets to improve your gut health and they haven't worked, there's a good chance that your digestive challenges can be chalked up to plant compounds – which is precisely why you picked up this book. This topic is pretty complex, and we want to give you a pretty thorough explanation, so let's make this a chapter of its own!

Chapter 2:

Plant Compounds

Jeff, a 28-year-old software developer, was the epitome of a modern professional juggling a demanding career and a flourishing social life. Jeff would wake up early each morning to get a workout in before hopping on the subway to downtown, where his office was located. After putting in 10-12 hours of hard work each day, Jeff would meet up with some friends after work to grab a bite to eat, have a drink, and head home to relax before waking up to do it all over again. To those around Jeff, he had it all going on. He was good-looking, funny, brilliant, and always seemed to be in a great mood. However, behind closed doors, Jeff's life was dominated by a less talked about struggle. Each meal he consumed led him down a path of discomfort, marked by persistent bloating, constipation, and the unpredictable disturbances of irritable bowel syndrome (IBS).

Jeff, like many, turned to the vast world of online health advice for answers. The consensus seemed clear and convincing: a diet rich in plants and especially fiber was the golden ticket to better digestive health. He learned that the gut was full of bacteria that needed to be fed with plants to thrive and that plants were the easiest foods to digest, which at the time sounded great given the constant discomfort Jeff was experiencing after eating. With a newfound sense of hope, Jeff revamped his diet to include an array of fruits, vegetables, whole grains, and legumes, anticipating a turn for the better.

Jeff's response to this dietary shift was unpredictably paradoxical. Rather than alleviating his symptoms, Jeff's high-fiber, plant-heavy diet seemed to amplify his digestive woes. The bloating became more pronounced, constipation more stubborn, and his IBS symptoms more erratic.

While this was discouraging to Jeff, he was honest with himself in understanding that while his diet was plant-based, it was far from clean. He often found himself opting for processed packaged foods with a plant-based label slapped on it. Jeff assumed he just needed to go a little harder with his plant-based approach: the results....absolutely no difference in his digestive distress.

One day during a lunch break, Jeff shared his frustrations with a colleague, we'll call him Andy, who happened to be a bit of a nutrition buff. Andy had actually just finished up the Carnivore Keto Cut program, a program created by Chris back in 2017 that helped people use a carnivore diet to reduce body fat percentage and gain muscle (yeah, carnivore can help with that, too!) Andy listened thoughtfully, then offered a different perspective. "It's not always about eating more plants and fiber. I've been following carnivore for four months now, and my digestion is better than it has ever been," he explained. Andy also shared that he had heard that a lot of people were seeing success using the carnivore diet for autoimmune and digestive disorders (though there was less info about this back then).

Jeff was skeptical but intrigued. In his initial research, he saw a lot about how meat was hard on the digestive system, plus he had been told his whole life that eating too much of it was bad for his heart. Regardless, Jeff was desparate and decided that it was worth a shot. Due to his preconceived notions about meat, though, he decided just to dip his toe in and started reducing certain plant foods and introducing more meat. His concern about red meat led to him eating more chicken and turkey than steak, but still, he gave it a shot.

Within a few days, Jeff noticed that some of his symptoms had gone away. He was feeling less constipated and bloated, and his IBS symptoms, though not completely gone, had gotten far more tolerable. Jeff was pretty pumped with his results.

One day after work, Jeff met up with some of his friends at their favorite plant-based restaurant in downtown Los Angeles. Since Jeff's symptoms were quite a bit better, he didn't think much about what he was ordering and decided to opt for a plant-based burger consisting of a blend of different beans, sweet potato, and quinoa with a side of broccolini. Later that night, when Jeff got home, he started to feel something rumbling in his gut. Shortly after, he found himself on the toilet with debilitating stomach pain and intense diarrhea, symptoms that he was all too familiar with.

Jeff was pretty demoralized by this setback. Had all that he had done with his diet been washed away by this one meal? Was he back at square one with the digestive discomfort he was so desparate to get rid of?

The next day, Jeff woke up feeling a little better but still not as good as he had been feeling. When he got to work that day, he decided to share what had happened to him with his friend Andy since it seemed like Andy was always looking for a reason to talk about how much he hated the plant-based diet movement. Andy, after making a few snide remarks about how silly he thought plant-based burgers were, gave Jeff a suggestion. "Maybe it's time you try full carnivore."

Jeff was still skeptical of the idea of eating an all-meat diet. After all, how could this be healthy, given all the saturated fat and cholesterol contained in meat? Despite this skepticism, Jeff remembered that eating fewer plants and more meat had definitely helped reduce his symptoms, and all he wanted was to go on with his life, living like a normal person. Jeff replied to Andy's suggestion with, "Who was that guy on Instagram you did the program with?"

Jeff reached out to me (Chris) at the end of 2017 and gave me a rundown of all that he was experiencing with his digestive discomfort. At the time, I was more plugged into the use of the carnivore diet for body composition and hormone regulation, but I had heard some anecdotes on social media and podcasts of people using the diet to improve their digestive health, so I told him that I thought it was worth a try and shared with him all of the carnivore resources I had at the time.

Despite his skepticism, Jeff jumped full into the carnivore diet this time. In fact, Jeff had some of the best adherence to the diet that I had ever seen. He was clearly motivated to make a change and defeat these digestive woes once and for all.

I checked in with Jeff weekly to see how he was adapting to the diet. After troubleshooting some initial complications like muscle cramps and trouble sleeping (we'll talk more about these later), Jeff told me that he was noticing a significant shift. Within a couple of weeks, what was left of his relentless bloating began to subside, and constipation eased. After about a month, his IBS symptoms became less frequent, and after two months, they were completely gone!

It's now been a couple of years since I have spoken with Jeff, but the last I knew, he was actually able to start incorporating certain plants back into his diet without the crippling digestive discomfort he had experienced before. Through reintroducing plants, Jeff found that there were certain plants that would cause slight flare-ups (though nothing like he felt before). Through analyzing which foods Jeff would experience discomfort from, we found that it was oxalates that he was most sensitive to. We'll get into these unique compounds in a bit.

I'm so happy that Jeff was able to get his life back with the carnivore diet. I hope today he is still experiencing the digestive peace that he reported to me back then. I am also grateful to Jeff because he was the first to show me the power of the carnivore diet in repairing gut health and eliminating digestive discomfort.

While Jeff's experience may sound unique to you, the truth is that his story is one of many similar stories. The "health halo" that has been placed around plants and the idea that a primarily plant-based diet is optimal for digestive health has been forced down our throats and has led many of us to overlook the potential harm that plant compounds can have on our gut health. This is precisely why it often catches people off-guard when they learn that plants may actually be at the root of their digestive issues. Why is that? The answer lies within some of the unique compounds found in plants.

So, What's the Deal with Plant Compounds?

Plants are made up of thousands of compounds that give them their unique biochemistry, many of which are often touted as being beneficial to health. Compounds like fiber and polyphenols are highlighted when talking about the health benefits of plants and are even isolated and put into supplements that we are recommended to take for benefits like improving gut health and combatting inflammation.

Again, we are not here to say that plants are all bad, but when you look at the research, you find that there are a variety of compounds in plants that can damage our digestive structure and trigger an immune response in the gut. Even compounds that are considered staples of a healthy diet in mainstream media, with fiber being the Taylor Swift of the plant-based community.

The Truth About Fiber

The "necessity" of fiber for a healthy gut is probably one of the most common arguments against a carnivore diet. We both remember much of our nutrition education in college was based around the idea that fiber is essential for optimal health and that the problem with our society's health was that a majority of the population isn't getting enough of it.

Today, if you visit any governing health and nutrition agency's website, you will frequently see recommendations for increasing fiber intake to reduce the risk of many chronic diseases ranging from type 2 diabetes and cancer to digestive disorders like IBS and constipation.

While there is no shortage of research supporting the benefits of fiber on digestive health, the research is actually much weaker than many realize and is mainly epidemiological (the weakest type of evidence). A lot of the studies reporting benefits from fiber are looking at the impact of switching from a Standard American Diet to a diet rich in fiber. We speculate that if you're consuming a diet rich in processed foods, sugar, and seed oils and you switch to food sources that contain more fiber, of course, you're going to get a bit healthier. You traded McDonald's for broccoli. Great choice! But that doesn't mean that fiber is necessarily the hero here.

The elementary explanation for the benefit of fiber is that it helps add bulk to your stool and increase the frequency of bowel movements. This is where the recommendation for increasing fiber intake when we are dealing with constipation comes from. The problem is that the research on fiber actually helping with constipation is less than clear.

One review of 5 studies covering nearly 200 patients failed to find significant evidence of fiber improving stool consistency, and there was no difference in painful bowel movements between groups that had more fiber and those that did not[1]. A study that divided subjects into either a high, low, or zero fiber diet found that the patients who completely stopped consuming fiber actually increased their bowel frequency from once every nearly four days to once every day. All of the individuals on the high-fiber diet continued to experience bloating, while 69% of the low-fiber participants and 100% of no-fiber participants completely eliminated their bloating[2].

The more scientific basis for the importance of fiber for our health is primarily based on the idea that fiber is broken down by gut microbes producing short-chain fatty acids (e.g., butyrate), which feed the cells of our gut lining while also contributing to gut microbial diversity. The belief is that without these prebiotic fibers from plants, we're starving the gut microbiome while the gut cells are also being starved of energy.

One important note to point out is that regardless of the benefit of butyrate, gut dysbiosis and gut inflammation impair the uptake of butyrate, so while fiber may serve someone with a healthy gut, someone who is trying to heal a gut issue may actually benefit from fueling their gut cells with alternative sources. More on that later in the book.

Yes, fiber can feed bacteria in the gut; the problem is that it doesn't differentiate between good and bad bacteria, which is why research has shown that fiber can promote the overgrowth of bad bacteria, potentially exacerbating conditions like small intestinal bacterial overgrowth (SIBO).

What about the idea that fiber improves the structural integrity of the gut? Diverticulitis, which is a digestive disorder characterized by the submucosa protruding from the outer muscular layer of the colon, is estimated to affect nearly 2.5 million people in the U.S. A study in over 2,000 patients found that the patients dealing with the worst degrees of diverticulitis were the ones consuming the most fiber [3,4].

The evidence against fiber doesn't just stop at digestive disorders, though. Research has also found that fiber can bind to certain minerals and affect their bioavailability or absorption. This includes minerals like zinc, calcium, magnesium, selenium, and iron [5].

It's important to understand that we are not necessarily saying that fiber is bad all of the time. The problem with fiber arises when gut dysbiosis and other digestive disorders are present. While many people do well with fiber, removing fiber from the diet has actually been shown to improve gut issues - eliminating bloating, constipation, and pain associated with digestion. For example, the study mentioned earlier found that subjects suffering from constipation saw improvements in their symptoms following the removal of fiber from their diet[2].

DO WE NEED FIBER?

Study Design:	Subjects suffering from constipation completely removed fiber from their diet
Results:	• Improvements in symptoms • Increase in bowel movements • Those who continued eating fiber showed no improvements
Conclusion:	Removing fiber from the diets of those suffering from digestive complications improves symptoms.

Citation: Ho et al 2012

Plant Defense Chemicals & Anti-Nutrients

Plants, though often perceived as passive and defenseless, possess a sophisticated arsenal of chemical defenses. These compounds, ingeniously woven into their very fabric, serve as the plant's shield and sword against a multitude of threats - from invading pathogens to herbivorous predators.

Plants produce a variety of defense chemicals, each with unique properties and mechanisms of action. Among these are the phytoalexins, which are dynamic compounds synthesized in response to microbial attacks. They emerge as part of the plant's immune response, rapidly accumulating at sites of infection or injury to ward off pathogens and pests.

Phytoalexins are synthesized rapidly in response to external threats and play a crucial role in the plant's immune system. Some well-known phytoalexins include:

- **Resveratrol:** Found in grapes, wine (especially red wine), peanuts, and some berries.
- **Salicylic Acid:** Commonly found in willow bark and is the precursor to aspirin.
- **Sulforaphane:** Found in cruciferous vegetables like broccoli, Brussels sprouts, and cabbage.
- **Pisatin:** Found in peas
- **Glyceollin:** Found in soybeans, particularly in response to fungal infection.
- **Capsidiol:** Found in pepper and tobacco plants

You may be familiar with some of these compounds, like resveratrol and sulforaphane, due to the typical promotion of their health benefits. However, the research in support of and against these molecules is less than clear.

What makes these compounds so alarming to us is that they are essentially natural pesticides. There has been a lot of talk about pesticide intake over the last couple of years, with a big emphasis placed on glyphosate. What many people don't realize is that 99+% of the pesticides we consume actually come from the plants themselves.

In a monumental scientific article written by Dr. Bruce Ames, it was estimated that Americans eat about 1.5g of natural pesticides per day, coming in over 40 different forms, depending on the specific contents of their diet[6]. More and more research is highlighting the fact that many of these compounds possess the ability to damage not only our digestive systems but our DNA as well.

Another group of plant compounds, antinutrients, while not primarily defense mechanisms, still indirectly protect plants. These compounds can deter herbivores by interfering with the digestion and absorption of nutrients, thus reducing the appeal of the plant as a food source.

If you have been following the constant and tiring debate around plant vs. animal-based diets, then you have likely heard some conversations around plant anti-nutrients. Often, the mainstream narrative around plant antinutrients is that they're an imaginary boogeyman that the carnivore community uses to fearmonger and turn people away from eating plants. While the fear-mongering may be true in some cases, these nutrients are real, and some people have issues with them.

The degree of tolerability to these antinutrients is highly dependent on the individual; some people may be able to deal with plant compounds better than others. If you have a compromised gut, however, you're likely more susceptible to these compounds. Let's break down some of these compounds so you can see what you are up against.

Oxalates

Oxalates, or oxalic acid, are compounds that occur naturally in many plant foods like nuts, kale, spinach, beans, chocolate, and several others. Interestingly, oxalates are not just found in food. They can also be produced by humans in the liver when we consume too much vitamin C, yeast, and fructose – all compounds that come from plants. The good news is that humans only produce a small amount of oxalates (much less than what plants provide to us) and possess natural detoxification pathways to eliminate these naturally occurring oxalates. The same may not be true for oxalates coming from plants.

In plants, oxalates are formed during photosynthesis and are used to bind to minerals like calcium, magnesium, and zinc to regulate the cellular concentration of these nutrients. The problem is that they also do this when we consume them, interfering with nutrient absorption and creating harmful compounds like calcium oxalate and iron oxalate. While most people can get rid of these compounds through stool and urine, some individuals have a sensitivity to these oxalates and, when consumed in large amounts, can experience gut issues[7] and even kidney stones if the compounds clump together and form crystals, needles, or stones in the bladder and gut wall[8]. In fact, 75% of all kidney stones are made from calcium oxalate.

Besides disrupting gut function, nutrient absorption, and possibly promoting kidney stones, research has also shown that an abundance of calcium oxalate can cause thyroid tissue damage and hypothyroidism[9].

If you notice that you feel bloated or inflamed after consuming a lot of plants, like Cynthia did, you may be sensitive to oxalates. Sensitivities can be due to a general digestive dysfunction, impaired gut function, or genetic alteration in a gene called SLC26A1, which is responsible for breaking down oxalate. Below is a list of the foods highest in oxalates.

Common Foods High in Oxalates

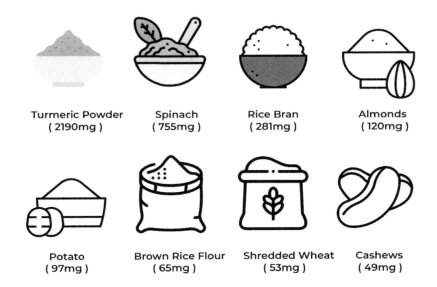

Turmeric Powder
(2190mg)

Spinach
(755mg)

Rice Bran
(281mg)

Almonds
(120mg)

Potato
(97mg)

Brown Rice Flour
(65mg)

Shredded Wheat
(53mg)

Cashews
(49mg)

Lectins

Lectins are proteins found in various plant-based foods, primarily seeds, legumes, tubers, and grains (e.g., wheat, potatoes, and beans) that have antinutrient properties. The problem with lectins is that they're "sticky." In scientific terms, this is known as agglutination, originating from the Latin word "agglutinate," which means "gluing to." Due to their stickiness, lectins can compromise the structure and function of the gut lining and work their way past the gut barrier to cause an autoimmune response[10].

Phytohemagglutinin (PHA) is a specific type of lectin found primarily in legumes and is highest in red and white kidney beans. PHA is known to be able to disrupt cell metabolism and is resistant to digestive enzymes, meaning it can pass through the G.I. tract intact. Research has shown that PHA can facilitate the growth of harmful bacteria like E.coli[11]. Even more concerning is that PHA can also bind to the surface of the gut, specifically goblet cells, causing damage that allows this bacteria in the gut to make contact with the gut epithelium and damage the mucosal layer. This triggers an immune response and the release of zonulin proteins, which exist to open those tight junctions between epithelial cells so that immune cells can get in the gut, fight off bad bacteria, and restore the health of the mucus layer.

Other studies have shown that lectins can bind to white blood cells, causing a release of inflammatory cytokines and potentially driving autoimmune conditions. Another lectin, Solanum Tuberosum Agglutinin (STA), found primarily in potatoes, can activate the immune system and the release of histamine, which in turn can lead to autoimmune symptoms like inflammation, swelling, itching, and hives[12].

Common Foods High in Lectins

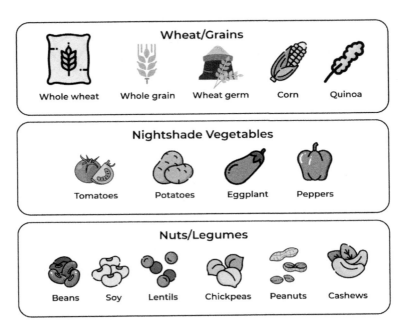

Gluten

You have probably heard of a lot about gluten and probably even know someone who either has celiac disease or is dealing with gluten sensitivity. Celiac disease is an autoimmune disorder that is triggered by gluten in genetically predisposed individuals, leading to impaired nutrient absorption, diarrhea, bloating, weight loss, anemia, and fatigue.

Gluten and celiac disease have been put through the mainstream health ringer because of how quickly the gluten-free movement was adopted. It became a joke when someone said they had celiac disease because it seemed like everyone had celiac disease, and how could this be if it's a genetic predisposition? Well, it turns out that a large portion of the population is what we call gluten-sensitive, creating another category called non-celiac gluten-sensitivity. These individuals do not possess the genetic alterations that cause gluten issues and thus do not have the same autoimmune damage that can occur in those with celiac. However, these individuals still experience a battery of digestive symptoms following gluten consumption.

So, what is gluten? Gluten is a family of proteins predominantly found in certain grains, such as wheat, barley, and rye. There are two primary components of gluten: gliadin and glutenin. Similar to lectins, gluten and, more specifically, gliadin is a major trigger of zonulin protein release, meaning they can interfere with the tight junctions in your gut, causing them to break open and contribute to leaky gut. Remember from Chapter 1, a leaky gut can lead to undigested food particles, bacteria, and other toxins leaking into the bloodstream, where they can trigger an autoimmune response and, thus, systemic inflammation. This effect is more apparent in celiac patients but can also affect those non-celiacs with gluten sensitivities. Research also indicates that gluten can negatively influence the composition of our gut microbiome, though the exact mechanisms here are not clear.

It's worth mentioning that for as many people who have issues with gluten, there are many people who seemingly do just fine with these proteins. However, it's possible that gluten is causing side effects that most people aren't drawing a connection to. For example, after going keto and carnivore for a while, Chris has noticed that when he lets gluten creep back into his diet, he experiences a flare-up in joint inflammation, knee pain, and struggles to recover from the gym. There are likely many others out there who are experiencing similar or unique side effects from gluten without realizing it.

Phytic Acid/Phytates

Phytic acid and phytates (the salt form of phytic acid) are natural substances found in plant seeds. In plants, phytic acid serves as a vital energy source for germination. It binds to essential minerals (such as calcium, magnesium, iron, and zinc) in the seed, making them available for the developing plant once it starts to grow. Phytic acid thus plays a crucial role in the plant's life cycle, ensuring that adequate nutrients are available during the critical stages of growth.

The human body does not seem to appreciate phytic acid as much. The primary issue with phytic acid is that it can bind to nutrients in the digestive tract and reduce absorption rates of key minerals like iron, zinc, magnesium, and calcium, potentially leading to nutrient deficiencies. For some people, diets high in phytate-rich foods can contribute to digestive discomforts like bloating and irregular bowel movements. The extent of these effects can vary widely among individuals.

Phytates are richest in whole grains like wheat, rice, barley, and oats, as well as nuts, seeds, legumes, and tubers. It is worth mentioning that you can reduce phytic acid from these food sources by soaking, sprouting, or fermenting.

Polyphenols

Polyphenols is a term that is generally associated with the benefits we get from plants, but it turns out that there is more to polyphenols than we realize. Polyphenols, often referred to as antioxidants, belong to a family of plant molecules with multiple phenol-like rings.

Maybe you have heard someone justify plant-based dieting by saying you should "eat the rainbow," referring to consuming plants from a broad spectrum of colors. These colors primarily come from polyphenols, which are rich in fruits like apples, grapes, and pomegranates, but also vegetables, nuts and seeds, and even whole grains. Included in the polyphenol family are popular and widely considered beneficial plant compounds like resveratrol, curcumin, and catechin. The role of pigmentation in plants is a defense mechanism against ultraviolet radiation, but some of these compounds offer other benefits, like resveratrol, which is found in the skins of grapes produced to ward off fungal attacks. All of this makes polyphenols a phytoalexin or defense chemical.

Polyphenols are often considered "natural" for humans, but it turns out that humans do not make these structures naturally. We only get them from plants. We also generally consider them beneficial to health, but it turns out that most of the research around their benefits is from epidemiological studies, and of the interventional studies that exist, we do not see the same degree of benefit.

For example, research on curcumin finds that most of the benefit of these molecules is found in test-tube studies that use doses way higher than what is found in the human body following turmeric ingestion[13,14]. The research looking at realistic doses of curcumin does not show the same evidence. In fact, curcumin has actually been shown to increase inflammation, potentially due to its impact on antioxidant defense enzymes.

Interestingly, the body knows what is best, so it actually hardly absorbs curcumin and quickly detoxifies and eliminates any amount it does absorb. Many curcumin supplements will try to prevent this by adding piperine to enhance absorption, but do we really want this?

A subclass of polyphenols that gets a lot of attention are flavonoids, including popular compounds like anthocyanins and isoflavones, which are commonly found in blueberries, strawberries, and raspberries. While there is some evidence reporting benefits from these compounds, we have also seen that they can also act as endocrine disruptors because their structure closely mimics estrogen. Research has especially shown that isoflavones can act as endocrine disruptors[15,16,17,18], with high intakes being associated with reduced fertility in animals and with anti-luteinizing hormone effects in premenopausal women. Catechins and quercetin are two other flavonoids that are popularly recommended for their health benefits; however, catechins have been connected with thyroid issues in animal models, and quercetin can bind to estrogen receptors and interfere with the breakdown of estrogen.

Another subgroup of polyphenols is tannins, which are commonly found in tea, red wine, apples, berries, grapes, and nuts. Tannins are defense molecules that inhibit the digestive enzymes of animals eating them. Interestingly, ruminant animals have developed proteins in their saliva that bind to tannins and render them inactive. Unfortunately, humans did not get this same capability, so tannins can inhibit our digestive enzymes. Research has shown that tannins can specifically inhibit protein digestive enzymes like trypsin and amylase and fat enzymes like lipase. This means that if we consume tannins with high protein + fat foods, it is likely that we will struggle with digestion, which can result in a decrease in net protein utilization.

It is worth mentioning that the research is not definitive enough to say whether polyphenols are beneficial for our health or not. There is so much conflicting information, with plenty of studies showing both sides of the story. Even in the primal community, there are differing opinions, with experts like Dr. Paul Saladino saying you should avoid polyphenols and experts like Dr. Steven Gundry saying we should include them. For now, our stance is that if you are displaying impaired digestion and nutrient deficiencies, it's worth cutting out polyphenols, at least for some period of time, to allow your gut the rest it needs to repair.

Sugar in Plants

The boom in type 2 diabetes rates and the rise in popularity of low-carb dieting have together led many to realize that we need to be paying attention to our sugar intake. However, there is still this lingering argument that the only thing we should concern ourselves with is added sugar because the sugar that is found in plants is natural and, therefore, good for our health. As you have now seen with many other naturally occurring plant compounds, this might not be the case.

Limiting sugar intake can be beneficial to nearly everyone, but it can be particularly beneficial for individuals with digestive issues, especially those suffering from digestive issues related to bacterial overgrowth. Several pathogenic gut bacteria feed off of sugar, so sugar from any source, plants included, will only add more fuel to the fire. Refined carbs and sugar are obvious offenders, but FODMAPs are also culprits.

FODMAPs

FODMAP stands for "fermentable oligosaccharides, disaccharides, monosaccharides, and polyols," which, in plain terms, just means fermentable sugars. While some people do just fine with FODMAPs, the small intestines can't absorb these sugars very well, and they have the potential to aggravate the gut. This is why many people suffering from irritable bowel syndrome (IBS) and/or small intestinal bacterial overgrowth (SIBO) benefit from removing them from their diet and is a big reason why low FODMAP diets have become popular strategies for combatting digestive complications.

High FODMAP Foods

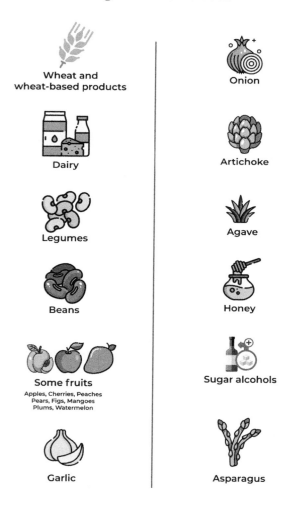

Wheat and wheat-based products

Dairy

Legumes

Beans

Some fruits
Apples, Cherries, Peaches
Pears, Figs, Mangoes
Plums, Watermelon

Garlic

Onion

Artichoke

Agave

Honey

Sugar alcohols

Asparagus

Sugar in Fruit:

When it comes to the natural sugar conversation, it is typically directed at the sugars in fruit, which we consider to be different and natural and give the green light to. It is true that the sugar found in fruit is different, but that doesn't necessarily mean that it's better.

Fruit can contain a variety of sugars, but the one that stands out the most is fructose. Fructose is still a sugar, meaning that it can still have the adverse effects that we see with all forms of sugar. In fact, research looking at the acute consumption of fructose found that this sugar can actually promote inflammation[19]. This study had subjects consume 50g of either glucose, fructose, or sucrose and found that consuming fructose led to the greatest increase in c-reactive protein, a common marker of inflammation.

There is also a lot of research showing that fructose can cause insulin resistance in the liver and even promote non-alcoholic fatty liver disease. It's important to note that a lot of this research is looking at high-fructose corn syrup, which is different and much worse than fructose from whole fruit, but it still highlights why we should be mindful of our fructose intake.

Certain fruits that are lower in sugar content, like berries, may be better tolerated, but the moral of the story is that it's probably a good idea to limit fruit consumption if you're dealing with digestive and autoimmune or inflammatory issues.

Agricultural Chemicals

Aside from the harmful compounds or anti-nutrients that can be found *inside* plants, there are also toxins found *outside* plants due to agricultural techniques like spraying fertilizers, pesticides, and herbicides. These chemicals can be very harmful to your health and further contribute to gut health issues.

Of the various agrochemicals out there, perhaps the most concerning is glyphosate, a compound more commonly known by the brand name RoundUp. Glyphosate is linked to a long list of health issues, with a particularly detrimental effect on gut health. Studies show that ingested glyphosate can kill off the beneficial bacteria in your gut and increase inflammation. Furthermore, due to the crucial role of microbes in the gut-brain axis, research suggests that glyphosate may promote neuroinflammation, potentially triggering neuropsychiatric conditions[20].

Shockingly, an NHANES study found that 81% of the US adult population has detectable levels of glyphosate in their body[21]. This herbicide is specifically used to kill pests that threaten genetically modified plants, such as corn and soybeans. That said, due to cross-contamination and the widespread use of RoundUp, this toxin can be detected in a wide range of plant foods.

EWG's 2021 "Dirty Dozen": the 12 MOST pesticide-contaminated produce items were:

1. Strawberries
2. Spinach
3. Kale, Collard & Mustard Greens
4. Peaches
5. Pears
6. Nectarines
7. Apples
8. Grapes
9. Bell & Hot Peppers
10. Cherries
11. Blueberries
12. Green Beans

I think it's safe to say that no amount of these agricultural chemicals is safe, but some individuals may not display as notable symptoms from their consumption. However, if you're dealing with digestive issues, then you would no doubt benefit from a break from these chemicals when you cut out plant foods on the carnivore diet.

The Hormetic Effect of Plant Compounds

It's worth mentioning that the anti-nutrients found in plants might not be all bad. While these compounds are associated with negative impacts on our health, recent research has suggested that some plant anti-nutrients may actually have a hormetic effect, which means that they can have a beneficial impact on health in small doses.

Hormesis is a biological phenomenon in which exposure to a low dose of a harmful substance or stressor can stimulate a positive response in an organism, leading to increased resistance to future stressors. Essentially, it's the idea that a little bit of "stress" can benefit you, as it stimulates the body's natural defenses and promotes adaptation and resilience. This concept has been observed in many different contexts, including exercise, exposure to cold or heat, and even certain toxins or substances in food. In the case of plant anti-nutrients, for example, low doses could stimulate the strengthening of the digestive lining following damage. That said, further research is still needed on this subject before we can be sure.

The hormetic effect of plant anti-nutrients is likely to occur because these compounds can trigger a stress response in the body, which in turn can stimulate cellular repair mechanisms and improve overall health. For example, some plant anti-nutrients have been shown to increase the activity of antioxidant enzymes in the body, which help to protect against oxidative damage and inflammation.

Studies have also suggested that plant anti-nutrients stimulate the growth of beneficial gut bacteria, which can have a positive impact on digestive health. For example, compounds such as resveratrol, found in grapes and red wine, and quercetin, found in onions and apples, have been shown to increase the abundance of beneficial bacteria such as Bifidobacterium and Lactobacillus.

With that being said, the overconsumption of these antinutrients is an issue, and if you're currently dealing with disrupted digestive health, even acute exposure could be problematic. For this reason, I recommend avoiding plant antinutrients while you're focusing on improving your gut health and, as I will get into during the reintroduction phase of the program, leveraging the hormetic effect to develop a more resilient gut once you have restored your gut health.

Chapter 3:

We Need Plants, Right?

Even though we just discussed the role plant toxins can play in digestive health. I bet you're still thinking that we need plants to survive, right? After all, we've been told since a young age how important it is to eat our vegetables, haven't we? "No dessert until you finish your broccoli." "If you want seconds, finish eating your peas and carrots first." While fat and processed carbohydrates have taken their fair share of criticism, no one dares to point a finger at vegetables – they're the shining star of the nutrition world. Aren't they? Especially with their robust nutrient density and superior nutrient absorption.

For most people, the concern around omitting plants from their diet is the belief that plants provide us with essential micronutrients that we can't get anywhere else, and cutting them out will lead to micronutrient deficiencies. Let's talk about why that's not the case.

Nutrient Absorption

Bioavailability is a term used to describe how much of a consumed substance is digested and enters the bloodstream, where the body can actually use it. If a food is highly bioavailable to humans, that means we can easily absorb and use most of the nutrients contained within that food. Conversely, if a food has a low bioavailability to humans, we poorly absorb most of the nutrients contained within that food.

While plants are indeed rich in various micronutrients, many of these micronutrients are poorly absorbed or have low bioavailability for humans. The micronutrients found in animal meat are a different story.

Research demonstrates that only *10-15%* of certain plant micronutrients can be absorbed by humans, while nearly *90%* can be absorbed from animal meat[1]. Vitamin A, for example, is 15-20x more bioavailable in meat compared to plant sources[2]. Plants also contain non-heme iron, which has demonstrated 3x *less* bioavailability compared to heme iron found in meat[3]. Then there's the food matrix, which describes the totality of nutrients in a food and how they interact during digestion. Many nutrients, such as vitamins D, E, K, and A, are fat soluble, meaning they're best absorbed by the body when consumed with dietary fat. While you'll rarely find sufficient fat in plant foods, it's almost guaranteed you'll have adequate fat for nutrient absorption in animal meat.

Another concern regarding the uptake of plant nutrients is those plant toxins I mentioned earlier. These anti-nutrients can actually interfere with the absorption of certain beneficial nutrients like folate, calcium, iodine, and zinc. You won't find these antinutrients in meat.

Ruminants to The Rescue

Now, you may be wondering what makes the nutrients found in animal meat better absorbed by humans compared to plants. The answer is that humans are carnivores/omnivores, and the animals that provide the red meat you eat on carnivore are herbivores. The most significant difference between the two is not just their food choices but their digestive systems.

Ruminant animals, which include cattle, sheep, goats, buffalo, deer, elk, giraffes, and camels, are a classification of animals with digestive systems that are much different from ours.

As opposed to our more simplistic digestive system, ruminants have four chambers in their stomachs: reticulum, rumen, omasum, and abomasum. When a ruminant animal eats plant material, it's only partly chewed before going into the rumen chamber of the stomach. The rumen chamber is rich with microorganisms that can break down plant material. Here, the partially chewed plant material is broken down into what is called "cud." Once an animal is full, it will continue to chew this cud to further break down the material before passing it off into the next three compartments of their digestive system: the reticulum, omasum, and their true stomach, the abomasum.

Interestingly, while it appears that these ruminant animals are on a low-fat, high-carb/fiber diet, the unique digestive tract actually allows them to ferment almost all plant matter into short-chain fatty acids, which go to the liver to form monounsaturated and saturated fats that are essential to the health and function of the animal.

This process is often referred to as "nutrient upcycling" because these ruminants can convert plant-based nutrients, largely inaccessible to humans, into forms that we can readily absorb. What is even more fascinating and important from an environmental process is that ruminants can even do this with waste products like corn husks, bean stalks, and orange peels. Again, here is a summary of how ruminants transform nutrients:

- **Unique Digestive System:** Ruminants have a specialized stomach divided into four compartments: the rumen, reticulum, omasum, and abomasum. The rumen acts as a fermentation vat where microbes break down fibrous plant materials like cellulose, which humans cannot digest.
- **Microbial Fermentation:** Within the rumen, a diverse community of bacteria, protozoa, and fungi work synergistically to ferment plant matter. This process converts complex carbohydrates into volatile fatty acids, which the animal then absorbs and uses as energy sources.
- **Synthesizing Essential Nutrients:** Ruminant microbes can also synthesize essential nutrients, including B vitamins and vitamin K2, from plant materials. These nutrients are vital for human health and are lacking in non-animal food sources.
- **High-Quality Protein Production:** The protein that ruminants get from plants is not complete but due to the digestive function of these animals, ruminant meat and milk are complete, containing all essential amino acids necessary for human health.
- **Filtering Agricultural Chemicals:** The digestive system of ruminant animals also allows them to file out agricultural chemicals, preventing them from finding their way into our diets when we eat ruminant meat

The point here is that humans don't have this same digestive system and thus cannot utilize plant-based foods in the same way. Our digestive systems are better designed to digest animal-based products and absorb the nutrients contained within them.

Ruminant Digestion

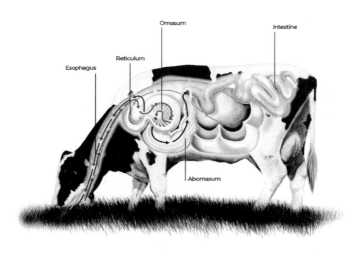

This is a big reason why we recommend ruminant animals as the primary food source for carnivore dieting. Pigs and chickens do not have these same digestive capabilities. Pork, while it can be nutrient dense, is very difficult to find quality sourcing for. Pigs will eat anything, and many producers take advantage of this by feeding them low-quality food. Since pigs aren't ruminants, they're unable to upcycle nutrients and filter toxins to the degree ruminants can. Poultry is also okay to eat, but it's typically much lower in nutrients, often fed soy, and again lacks the ability to upcycle and filter like ruminants can. All of this means that these sources of meat are not as nutrient-dense, and the plant compounds and agricultural chemicals fed to these animals may be able to make their way into our diets. Not ideal for gut restoration.

This doesn't mean that you have to completely avoid poultry and pork on carnivore. In fact, we recommend including it here and there to switch things up and prevent yourself from getting bored. Our suggestion is, if you want to ensure that you're getting the nutrients you need to repair your gut and perform optimally in your day-to-day life, we think it is best to have at least 80% of your protein coming from red meat/ruminants.

Sourcing Meat

Meat sourcing is a heavily debated topic in the carnivore space, with different camps holding different opinions. We're going to fearmonger a bit here, but we'll help you understand why.

We think food quality is important. we know not everyone wants to admit it, but there's a big difference between a grass-fed steak and a bunless burger cooked in vegetable oils from McDonald's. Let's look at why:

A recent review demonstrated that grass-fed cattle have a greater proportion of conjugated linoleic acid (CLA) and omega-3 fatty acids on a gram-per-gram basis4. CLA has been associated with improving insulin sensitivity and may aid in muscle maintenance and weight loss. Meanwhile, Omega 3's play a variety of important roles throughout the body, including cell membrane development, neuronal development, and reducing inflammation. Additionally, these researchers also found that grass-fed cattle had elevated precursors for vitamins A and E, and the potent antioxidant glutathione compared to grain-fed.

The other concern with grain-fed meat is the actual grain that is being eaten. Under conventional agriculture standards, the grain being fed to these cows is likely covered in agricultural chemicals. As we mentioned earlier, there is some potential for cows to filter out these chemicals, but we think it would be silly to think these chemicals don't have some sort of impact on the animal.

That said, we must admit that the research on the health benefits of grass-fed vs. grain-fed meat is rather conflicting. While some reviews (like the one mentioned above) make a clear case for grass-fed cattle, other studies demonstrate little difference. For this reason, we always tell people that you should opt for what you can afford. Grain-fed meat is better than no meat. Of this, we are certain.

Aside from human health, the environmental impact of your meat is another reason to consider your source. We won't exhaust this topic in this book since others have done a much better job (check out the book Sacred Cow by Robb Wolf and Dianna Rodgers). But to leave a quick note, know that grass-fed and finished meat tends to come from farms following more environmentally friendly animal agriculture practices. Ruminant animals are meant to live on vast acres of land, munching on the greenery provided by that land. When they do this, they also excrete urine and feces into the soil, which is essential to the microbial diversity of the soil the animals are living on. Animals living in feed lots are likely fed mono-crops sprayed with chemicals while also excreting vast amounts of feces and urine due to the number of animals living in such tight quarters. Neither of which is optimal for the environment.

Store-bought grass-fed/finished meat can be expensive, so we recommend checking your local farmer's market or searching your area for local farmers selling meat. When you do this you not only get a higher quality source of meat that's more environmentally friendly, but you also support your local economy. To save even more on grass-fed meat, you can look at buying in bulk by ordering a full cow or even a cow-sharing program where you split a whole cow with other friends. When you buy in bulk, you will find that the average cost per pound of meat is much more affordable.

For those who live in areas without easy access to local farms, services like Nose-to-Tail and Force of Nature are great ways to get quality beef shipped to your door!

Specific Nutrient Absorption Differences

Below is a breakdown of many key nutrients and how much of them is absorbed from different food sources.

(100g)	Blueberries	Kale	Beef	Beef Liver
Calcium	6.0 mg	72 mg	11 mg	11 mg
Phosphorus	12 mg	28 mg	140 mg	476 mg
Potassium	77 mg	228 mg	370 mg	380 mg
Iron	0.3 mg	0.9 mg	3.3 mg	8.8 mg
Zinc	0.2 mg	0.2 mg	4.4 mg	4.0 mg
Vitamin A	None	None	40 IU	53,400 IU
Vitamin D	None	None	Trace	19 IU
Vitamin E	0.6 mg	0.9 mg	1.7 mg	.63 mg
Vitamin C	9.7 mg	41 mg	None	27 mg
Niacin	0.4 mg	0.5 mg	4.0 mg	17 mg
Vitamin B6	0.1 mg	0.1 mg	.07 mg	.73 mg
Vitamin B12	None	None	1.8 mcg	111 mg
Folate	6 mcg	13 mcg	4.0 mcg	145 mcg

Source: https://chriskresser.com/got-digestive-problems-take-it-easy-on-the-veggies/

Vitamin A

The form of vitamin A that humans absorb is retinol. Plants provide vitamin A in the form of carotenoids, which must be converted to retinol. This conversion rate is, unfortunately, very low. Animal foods, on the other hand, provide retinol directly – no conversions required. This is precisely why vitamin A from animal sources has been shown to be far more bioavailable compared to plant sources[5]. As mentioned earlier, research shows that animal sources of vitamin A are 15-20x more bioavailable than plant sources—one of the many reasons why plant-based dieters are often deficient in this nutrient.

Vitamin D

Humans absorb vitamin D as D3, which we can get from sunlight and animal foods. The form of vitamin D in plants is D2, which must be converted to D3 in the body. Vitamin D3 is significantly more bioavailable than D2[6], and there's evidence that, compared to omnivores, vegans have lower vitamin D levels, especially during winter months when the sun is taken out of the equation[7].

Vitamin K

The type of vitamin K that has the most biological activity is K2. This is only found in animal foods, with the exception of some fermented foods that most people aren't eating regularly, like natto (fermented soybeans....with all their plant toxins). Plants, on the other hand, contain K1, which is converted to K2 in negligible amounts and doesn't have the same beneficial effects that K2 does on the health of our bones, arteries, and brain[8].

B Vitamins

Of the B vitamins, B12 is the most well-known to be lacking in vegan or vegetarian diets because it's primarily found in animal foods. Plant-based dieters are at a much higher risk of developing B12 deficiencies, the consequences of which are quite serious. All other B vitamins are found in plant foods, including B1 (thiamin), B2 (riboflavin), B3 (niacin), B5 (pantothenic acid), B6 (pyridoxine), B7 (biotin), and B9 (folate). However, some are found in greater abundance in animal foods, particularly B2 (riboflavin), and some have been shown to be more bioavailable when sourced from animals (e.g., B6)[9].

Iron

Plants contain a form of iron called non-heme iron, which is well known to be less absorbed than heme iron found in meat. Heme iron is also the form of iron that the human body uses[10]. Vegans and vegetarians have a higher prevalence of iron deficiencies[11],which can provoke many symptoms, including fatigue, muscle weakness, and even depression.

Zinc

Zinc comes primarily from animal foods. It can be found in some plant foods (e.g., legumes, grains, nuts, and seeds), but these same plant foods are high in phytic acid, which inhibits the absorption of zinc[12], making it very difficult to reach adequate zinc levels on a plant-based diet.

Omega-3 Fatty Acids

Omega-3 fatty acids are essential, meaning we can not produce them and must obtain them through the diet. These nutrients are absolutely crucial to brain health. The biologically active forms of omega-3 are EPA and DHA, found specifically in animal foods. The form of omega-3 in plant foods is alpha-linolenic acid (ALA), which converts to EPA at rates of about 5-10% and DHA 2-5%[13].

ALA is the source of omega-3 fats for ruminant animals, but again, these ruminants come to the rescue and take ALA from the plants they are eating, convert it to EPA/DHA for us, and store it in their muscle meat, where we can have better access to a superior source of omega-3 fatty acids.

Cholesterol & Saturated Fat

Cholesterol and saturated fat have long been demonized as the cause of many health issues, particularly cardiovascular disease. Later in the book, we'll go over why this isn't the case and how our society has come to this conclusion.

The truth is that both cholesterol and saturated fat are *essential* to human health. They're necessary for the production of key hormones and even the structure and functioning of our brain. Plant foods do not contain significant amounts of these nutrients, and despite what the mainstream media says, this is not a reason to eat more plants and fewer animals!

Essential Amino acids

There are nine essential amino acids that humans must obtain through diet, and all 9 of them are found in animal foods. That's why animal foods are referred to as being a "complete source of protein." In contrast, plant foods are incomplete proteins and are missing certain key amino acids, requiring food combinations if you want to get all nine essential amino acids. It goes further than this, though. Remember, plant proteins are poorly absorbed and less bioavailable compared to animal proteins.

Meaning even if you were to consume the same amount of protein from plants as you were from animals, you would absorb less. Animal foods supply the highest quality and most bioavailable complete protein.

This information is reflected in the PDCAAS score of a food, which stands for Protein Digestibility Corrected Amino Acid Score. The PDCAAS score assesses:

1. The amino acid content of the food
2. How well those amino acids are digested and absorbed, given the food matrix

Unsurprisingly, animal proteins have significantly higher PDCAAS scores than plant proteins. For example, the PDCAAS score of an egg is 1.0 (which is the highest score available), while the PDCAAS of quinoa is 0.78. The PDCAAS score of beef is 0.92, While the PDCAAS score of lentils is 0.73[14,15].

Why Do We Even Recommend Eating Plants Then?

This is a great question. If we can't get the proper nutrients from plants that we need to survive and thrive, then why do so many people insist we eat plants? In addition to the dogma that's been ingrained in all of us since we were children, another great explanation can be found in an explanation from Dr. Georgia Ede that goes something like this: It may be that vegetables appear so healthy in all the epidemiological studies because of what they are not, and not because of what they are.

What Dr. Ede is saying is that many of the studies demonstrating the benefits of eating vegetables are likely looking at the wrong factors.

In most plant-based diet studies, prior to the intervention, subjects are consuming a typical Standard American Diet, or SAD, consisting of refined carbohydrates and ultra-processed foods. Again, swapping McDonald's out for broccoli is going to lead to improvements in health. But just because a diet is better than the horrible diet most of our society is consuming today, it doesn't mean that it's the optimal diet for a human to consume.

Chris experienced this phenomenon with his friend Josh, who was addicted to Taco Bell. One year, Josh finally decided to take Chris's advice and start cooking at home. As a New Year's resolution, he made it a challenge to avoid all fast food for at least one month. After about two weeks on his new "diet," Josh was feeling great and ready to take things a step further and decided to go full vegan. Josh responded really well to the vegan diet and continued to follow it for the rest of the year.

Unfortunately, after about ten months, things started to take a turn. With all of his renewed energy, Josh took up running in the spring, but by Fall, he found that his joints began to ache, and he could no longer muster the energy to beat his best times. He also noticed some hair loss, and although he had shed a significant amount of weight, around 30 pounds, he wasn't making any muscle gains at the gym.

When he came to Chris for some advice, the answer was clear: Josh wasn't getting enough protein.

The takeaway? Sure, Josh felt amazing getting off Taco Bell, but a plant-based diet wasn't the answer either - it was just a better option than fast food.

The truth is that most plant-based diets demonstrate improvements in the short term but, in the long term, demonstrate numerous side effects from nutrient deficiencies because we can't get the nutrients we need to survive and thrive from plant sources alone.

On paper, plants seem awesome; chock full of vitamins, minerals, amino acids, some healthy fats, seemingly the whole package. The problem is, as humans, we just can't access these nutrients very well.

Chapter 4:

Introduction to the Carnivore Diet

I (Chris) first heard about the carnivore diet back in 2016 when my friend Danny Vega told me about some of the success he had experienced on the diet. To be honest, I was really skeptical.

I had been studying keto for a little over two years at that point, so I was past the whole "meat is bad for you" concept (if you're not, don't worry, we will get to that soon), but eating meat is one thing. ONLY eating meat is an entirely different story.

Right around this same time, I came across the work of Dr. Shawn Baker, an avid carnivore dieter, and leader of the carnivore movement, and heard Dr. Jordan Peterson talk about his and his daughter Mikhaila's success using carnivore for autoimmunity and depression on the Joe Rogan Experience Podcast. This made my gears start to turn. I decided to give the diet a shot and see what all the hype was about.

Similar to my first adventure into ketosis, I made a lot of mistakes my first time on carnivore. I didn't prioritize food quality; I was likely consuming too much dairy, and I combined it with intermittent fasting, which can be a great strategy, but for me, it led to way too low of a calorie intake than what my body was demanding. Still, what I experienced on the diet was incredible.

My energy was insane. Even better than on keto. I noticed that the joint pain that had previously plagued my ankles and knees from years of basketball was alleviated in just a couple of weeks. And most relevant to this book, my digestive system started functioning way better. I was incredibly impressed.

Cynthia started learning more about carnivore when she started dealing with her own health complications. Shawn Baker's work also played a big role in introducing the diet to Cynthia, but at the time, she had not eaten mammalian meat in over 20 years! A big reason why she had some healthy skepticism around the diet as well.

Since those early years, a lot more research has come out, more doctors are now supporting the diet, and hundreds of thousands of anecdotes and success stories from the diet are now fueling the growing awareness of the carnivore diet's power.

While I was living in Austin, Texas, I used carnivore a lot. One of the most memorable to me was when I was writing the Keto Answers book because I found that carnivore was a great diet to boost productivity. The ease of following the diet, the energy and clarity boost I got, and, in particular, the lack of hunger allowed me to stay focused on writing for long stretches at a time.

During my time in Austin, I was also introduced to the concept of food quality, which we will get into later in this book. Understanding food quality led to more knowledge of food sourcing, which led to my carnivore diet looking even more ancestral and optimal.

To this day, we both eat a much more meat-centric diet and still use the carnivore diet as a tool when trying to achieve specific goals that carnivore is best suited for. That's the purpose of this book: to show you how to use the carnivore diet as a tool for, in this case, resetting your digestive system and optimizing your gut health.

What is Carnivore?

The carnivore diet, as its name suggests, is an animal-based diet. By animal-based, we mean you eat animals and food products that come from animals. Check out the food pyramid below:

Carnivore Food Pyramid

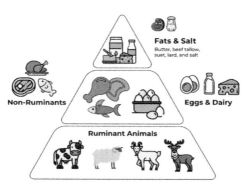

Right out of the gate, this may seem a bit extreme because of the societal notion that "eating your vegetables" is required for good health. As we covered a bit in the last chapter and as we will continue covering throughout the book, this isn't necessarily the case.

While my first introduction to the carnivore diet took place in 2016, the history of this way of eating dates back much further, humans have consumed a primarily carnivorous diet for a significant portion of our existence. Early humans were hunter-gatherers, and most of their diets consisted of meat and fish, supplemented by occasional fruits, vegetables, and nuts when available. In fact, archaeological studies have found evidence of animal bones and stone tools used for hunting and butchering as far back as 2.6 million years ago. Indigenous cultures like the Inuit, the Masai, and the Hadza have also traditionally consumed all or mostly meat. All of this changed when humans developed agricultural prowess, and diets slowly started shifting more and more plant-based.

Throughout history, nutrition experts have gone back and forth on meat. Similar to what we hear today, some experts say to avoid meat at all costs, while others say to eat nothing but meat.

In the 19th century, a carnivore diet started to gain traction when Scottish doctor James Salisbury (I know what you're thinking…) recommended an "all-meat diet" because he believed it could cure many ailments, including constipation and tuberculosis.

Despite the strong push to demonize meat, a carnivore way of eating continued to gain traction in the 20th century when bodybuilders and athletes found that this high-protein diet was an excellent strategy for supporting muscle growth and exercise performance.

Today, with the help of top health experts like Dr. Shawn Baker and Mikhaila Peterson (now Fuller), carnivore continues to explode as more and more individuals are finding a ton of success in losing weight, managing autoimmune diseases, and improving gut health.

Red Meat vs. White Meat vs. Seafood on Carnivore

We've established that carnivore is a diet consisting of eating primarily meat; however, there are a ton of choices for meat. You can opt for red meat coming from ruminants like cows, bison, and elk. You can opt for white meat like pork, chicken and turkey. Or you could opt for seafood ranging from fresh to salt water and even shellfish.

From a general sense, opting for any combination of these meats is likely fine. If the goal is choosing what is optimal, then the focus should be placed on red meat. If you recall from the last chapter, ruminant animals have unique digestive systems that allow them to convert and store nutrients in versions that are more easily absorbed by the human body. They are also great at filtering out environmental toxins that can also contribute to poor health and digestive distress. Pigs, chickens, turkeys, and fish do not have this same capability.

For this reason, we recommend sticking primarily to red meat. Especially if you are following carnivore for complete gut restoration. This does not mean complete avoidance of these other sources of meat, especially since the variety can help with adherence. But as we will cover in Chapter 8, there is good reason to avoid these sources during the initial elimination phase of the Carnivore Reset protocol.

Dairy on Carnivore

Dairy is a very polarizing topic in the health space. On the one hand, you'll often hear people flag the fact that we're the only known species that drinks milk from another animal. This camp claims that consuming milk or milk products from other animals offers little to no benefit for us as humans. On the other hand, there are those who note that dairy offers a highly bioavailable source of nutrition, which humans have consumed for centuries. Even within the ancestral community, you'll hear both sides of the story. With all of this back-and-forth, It's pretty confusing to figure out where to stand.

Dairy is an animal-based food so therefore it is considered carnivore. But whether or not you consume it is dependent on many factors. One of the big reasons why this topic is debated so much is because there are vastly different forms of diary. Dairy can be consumed raw, sold directly from a farmer, or pasteurized and homogenized from a store. It can also be stripped of some of its key macro and micronutrients and have other less optimal ones added. The result is drastically different forms of dairy within our food landscape.

The truth is that most store-bought dairy offers much less benefit to our health. Let's take milk, for example. When milk is processed as heavily as it is to be approved to be on grocery store shelves, it offers little nutritional benefit outside of the macronutrients and calories it contains. The pasteurization process removes the beneficial bacteria found in milk, further dampening the potential benefit. When you get to the low-fat and 2% milk, you'll find that fat, one of the most beneficial components of dairy, is removed and often replaced with sugar.

Contrary to conventional belief, this is not a very beneficial trade-off for our health. Other forms of store-bought dairy can be even worse. Most yogurts are loaded with added sugar and often contain seed oils.

The main reason why you would consider avoiding dairy on carnivore or any other diet is because of dairy intolerances. However, as you may be able to infer when it comes to dairy intolerances, most people are experiencing the intolerances from store-bought dairy, making it hard to say if their intolerance is actually to dairy or the processed junk at the grocery store.

Of course, there are individuals who actually are sensitive to dairy with the culprits being the sugars (lactose and d-galactose) and the proteins (casein and albumins) found in dairy. Interestingly, case reports demonstrate that even for these individuals, the issue may be in the processing of the milk.

When milk is pasteurized, the digestive enzymes responsible for aiding in dairy digestion, especially lactase, are filtered out of the milk, resulting in a final product that's harder to digest. Many individuals with lactose intolerance actually find that they can drink raw dairy with no issues but struggle with store-bought dairy. Regardless, for the purpose of this reset, we recommend keeping dairy limited, especially in the early stages. Dairy can be brought back during the reintroduction phase if well tolerated. We'll talk more about that in Chapter 8.

If you are not dealing with severe digestive complications and do not notice any issues when you consume dairy, then it can be a fine addition to a carnivore diet. It's important to focus on the source, though. The best dairy you'll be able to find is raw dairy, but sourcing it isn't easy because most states have outlawed the sale of raw dairy directly to the consumer. Interestingly, many farmers' markets have found workarounds for this by labeling the dairy "not for human consumption" or for pet consumption only." If you're interested in trying it, go covert and bring a dog with you to the market.

If you don't have access to a farmer's market, you can make store-bought dairy work. Look for full-fat versions and check the ingredients to ensure no sugar or seed oils have been added. You can also look for A2 dairy, a variation of dairy containing a different type of casein protein, one of the proteins people are sensitive to in dairy. A2 is typically better tolerated than A1, and A1 is the version that's more closely linked with gut and immune disorders. You can tell the difference by looking at the milk container because A2 dairy is always labeled—something to keep in mind during the reintroduction phase of the Carnivore Reset protocol.

You can also consider fermented dairy like yogurt, aged cheese, and kefir. Fermented dairy contains several beneficial probiotic bacteria that can help repopulate your gut microbiome. It's also a source of K2, an essential nutrient for maintaining healthy bones. For this reason, we'll be recommending fermented dairy in the reintroduction phase after the reset.

Ultimately, whether you include dairy or not will be based on your own tolerance. If you are following the elimination protocol in this book, we recommend avoiding it, but if you feel confident that you don't have an aversion to dairy, feel free to stick with it. Just be aware of the type of dairy you're consuming and how your body responds to different sources to identify which is best.

Eggs on Carnivore

Eggs are also an animal-based food, making them carnivore-friendly; however, eggs can also cause digestive issues in some individuals. Here is what you need to know.

There can be several causes for egg sensitivities, but the most common is the two proteins found in eggs: albumin and ovomucoid. Both of which are found in the egg white. If these proteins are not properly digested, they can cause digestive symptoms such as bloating, gas, and diarrhea.

Another reason for sensitivity to eggs could be the way they're prepared. Most eggs bought at a restaurant will be cooked in seed oils, which could produce gut discomfort if you're already struggling with a damaged gut. It's also possible that the food the chicken was fed will affect your sensitivity. Soy, which is commonly used in chicken feed, is loaded with anti-nutrients that can impair digestion and inhibit the absorption of key nutrients. You will likely only have a problem with this aspect of eggs if you have more severe digestive complications.

While all of this may make eggs sound like a food to be avoided, that's definitely not the case. In fact, eggs are one of the most nutrient-dense foods we can consume. An egg provides all of the nutrients required to grow life, you better believe it can do a lot for us as well!

Again, if you are following the Carnivore Reset protocol for severe digestive issues, we recommend removing eggs from the first two weeks to allow your digestive system to rest and reset before reintroducing this nutritional powerhouse. We will talk more about this in chapter 8.

Spices on Carnivore

Who would have ever thought that spices would be a topic of debate in nutrition? Carnivore has definitely made this the case. Many carnivore purists will also say that a true carnivore diet does not include spices because spices are of plant origin and contain compounds like histamines or salicylates that could trigger a digestive reaction if you have an underlying condition. We think there is a case to be made for this. Certainly, some spices, like black pepper or chili powder, can irritate the gut lining, which is counterproductive to the goal of allowing complete digestive rest and repair.

Again, if you are just following carnivore for general benefits and are free of major digestive issues, spices are likely fine and can make a great addition to help keep your diet interesting and flavorful. As we will cover in Chapter 8, for the more intense experience of the Carnivore Reset, we will remove these spices for the first couple of weeks.

Macros & Calories on Carnivore

If you have ever followed a weight loss (or gain) diet, then you're likely familiar with macros and calories. Macros, or macronutrients, are the major components that make up food consisting of protein, fat, carbs, and fiber.

Many diets, like keto, offer a specific set of macronutrient ranges to adhere to when following the diet. Even in diets like keto, these ranges are often too rigid and fail to take into consideration the unique needs of the individual following the diet. Regardless, on carnivore, there is no strict set of macros that make a diet carnivore. Instead, macros and calories should be tailored to your unique needs to help you reach your goal.

In Chapter 8, we will talk more about macro and calorie recommendations for this program, but it's worth pointing out here that we believe most individuals can operate just fine simply focusing on what to eat and what not to eat on carnivore without having to deal with the constant stress of tracking macros and calories.

Organ Meat

If you are like most people, the idea of eating organ meat immediately triggers the thought, "Yuck, there's no way I'm eating that." Before you count it out, give us a chance to make a case for this incredibly beneficial food source.

Back in the hunter and gatherer era, each aspect of the animal was utilized, not just the muscle and fur, but the organs too! In fact, organ meat was considered a delicacy. Many ancestral tribes saved organs for the warriors and, in some cases, even the children to ensure proper nutrition for optimal growth. Even amongst predator animals, organs are prized. When a pack of wolves hunts an animal, the alpha wolf has first pickings, and guess what they go for first – the liver!

As humans, we typically just eat the muscles of animals and neglect the organ meat. Not only is this wasteful, but we're getting rid of high-quality protein sources that are incredibly rich in micronutrients.

While the exact nutrient content will differ slightly from source to source and animal to animal, in general, organ meats are a great source of:

•   Protein

- Vitamin B12
- Vitamin A
- Folate
- Choline
- Selenium and Iron

The most common types of organ meats include liver, heart, and kidneys. The most common animal sources include cow, lamb, goat, pork, and chicken. Of course, we recommend sticking with ruminant sources. Let's do a quick breakdown of each of the organs and why you should consider implementing them into your carnivore diet:

Liver

Liver is one of the more popular organ meats because it happens to be the most nutrient-dense option. A 3.5-ounce serving of beef liver contains 25 grams of protein and over 1300% of the RDI for Vitamin B12. Additionally, liver is also high in iron, copper, vitamin A, and niacin. Collectively, these nutrients can reduce oxidative stress (vitamin A) and provide a cardio-protective effect (vitamin B).

Heart

The heart is typically known for being one of the tastier organ meats. Like the liver, the heart is a great source of vitamin B12. Additionally, the heart has >50% of the RDI for riboflavin.

Furthermore, what makes the heart special (especially cow heart) is that it contains coenzyme Q10 (CoQ10), which helps generate energy and functions as an antioxidant, protecting the cells from free radicals and oxidative stress. Low levels of CoQ10 are linked with heart disease, diabetes, and cancer. Research has shown that increasing CoQ10 intake can improve exercise performance and may even reduce the severity of migraines by improving mitochondrial function[1,2].

Kidneys

Kidneys are rich in vitamin B12 and selenium. Cow kidneys have over 200% of the RDI for selenium. Selenium appears to improve blood flow, which leads to a variety of beneficial downstream effects, including improved cardiovascular function, immune function, metabolism, and antioxidant capacities.

Other Organs

Other organ meats include the intestines (tripe), tongue, brain, and testicles but these are often less consumed. To be honest, we don't eat these sources of organs because we have to draw the line somewhere. Feel free to do the same.

The Source Matters

When it comes to meat, the source does matter, and it may matter even more for organ meat. Organ meats are regarded as safe for human consumption, but opting for grass-fed/finished will ensure you're getting the highest quality. Animals raised in cleaner, more natural environments are less likely to accumulate toxins in their organs. This is crucial as organs can be a site of toxin detoxification and sometimes accumulation if the animal is exposed to a high level of pollutants or harmful feed. Check out the resource section at the end of the book to learn more about sourcing quality meat.

Cooking Organ Meat

We will say we're not experts in this area and are still working on perfecting our organ meat cooking skills. Most times, Chris just cuts raw organs into small pieces and swallows whole to avoid experiencing too much of the taste and because when it's raw, the meat may offer more nutrition. There are some inherent risks from doing this, which is why we're not recommending you do the same. Generally speaking, it seems like the more you cook organ meat, the worse the taste is, which is why we recommend not overcooking.

One great hack for organ meat is using organ meat blends. Organ meat blends are ground meat blends containing a combination of muscle meat and typically liver and/or heart. Depending on where you live, you can get this at your local farmer's market, but if not, Force of Nature is our go-to source. We love these blends because you can easily incorporate them into stew and other recipes to help mask the taste.

At the end of this book, we'll provide a few organ meat recipes to help improve the taste of this food. But we also think it is worth mentioning that maybe it's okay if all of the food we eat isn't absolutely delicious. Sometimes, the benefits are worth the discomfort of consuming something that doesn't taste the best.

Variations of the Carnivore Diet

As you can see, there is some nuance to this seemingly simple diet. This is why, as the diet has continued to grow in popularity, new ways of executing the diet have evolved. Here are a few common variations you may hear of:

- **Meat Only Carnivore:** Likely the most popular and least confusing variation of carnivore, only meat and typically primarily red meat are consumed. This is likely the best choice, at least at first, for individuals dealing with digestive distress and autoimmunity. But also, a lot of people work in a binary fashion, where they like the guessing game to be taken out of the equation - it's a simple "yes" or "no." The meat-only carnivore diet works very well for these folks as well. The optimal version of this variation should include nose-to-tail eating, meaning organ meats are included.
- **Animal-Based Carnivore:** This variation of carnivore consists of eating only animal products, including fish, eggs, poultry, and dairy sources like cheese and butter if you so choose. If you get bored quickly with your food and like to mix things up but want to achieve most of the benefits of a meat-only carnivore diet, this version is for you.
- **95% Carnivore:** Many people following the carnivore diet tend to make exceptions and allow for non-carnivore oils like coconut oil or may even slide an occasional avocado, some blueberries, or honey in their diet. This is something we term as 95% carnivore. That 5% gives people a little wiggle room to play with some less toxic plant foods, which may translate to better compliance. This can be a great option for those not requiring as strict of an approach to experience the benefits of carnivore.
- **Cyclical Carnivore:** Consuming carnivore during the week but having fruits/vegetables and/or other non-carnivore foods on the weekend. Some people following this diet may even choose to eat carbohydrate cheat meals on the weekend. If you're going to do this, the best way is to stick to "cleaner" carb sources like root vegetables or low-glycemic fruit. This approach can be great for weight loss and to generally improve overall wellness however, if you are dealing with digestive complications, while this approach may provide benefits, it is not optimal and will likely be insufficient.

How to choose the right variation for you:
Choosing the right variation of carnivore will be dictated by your goals,

your food preferences, and your sensitivity to certain foods. For example, some people may want to have as much variety in their carnivore diet as possible, so they'll opt for the 95% or Animal-Based version of the diet. Others may be sensitive to certain animal-based products like eggs or dairy and thus will be required to follow a more strict, meat-only carnivore diet.

Because you're on a journey to heal your gut, we recommend starting somewhere between the Meat Only and Animal-Based variations, at least for your healing phase, but we'll get into that a bit later in the book.

The Carnivore/Keto Overlap

If you've heard of the carnivore diet, it's likely that you're also familiar with the keto diet and may be wondering what the difference is. Carnivore and keto actually have a lot of overlap. The ketogenic diet is followed with the clear intention of elevating blood ketone levels and thus inducing a state of ketosis where fats and ketones have taken the reins from glucose as the body's primary fuel. This is accomplished by dramatically reducing dietary carbohydrates. The carnivore diet is essentially a zero-carb diet, meaning it also promotes ketosis without it even being the objective. We believe a lot can be gained by formulating your carnivore diet to be ketogenic for both health and practical reasons, and we have taken this into consideration when creating the protocol we will introduce in Chapter 8.

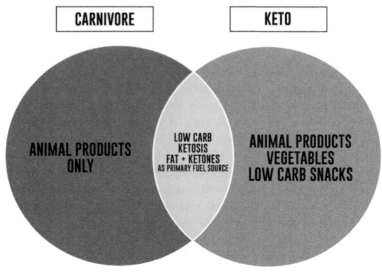

Isn't a keto diet good enough?

Many people can achieve a ton of success with keto, especially if the goal is restoring metabolic health, weight loss, stabilizing blood sugar, increasing energy, and decreasing hunger. However, for some individuals, especially those dealing with autoimmune and gut complications, keto might not be enough. Between the increased number of "keto-friendly" processed foods and the vegetables often approved on this diet, individuals trying to optimize for gut health may find that it's best to cut out plant-based foods and stick to a meat-only or animal-based version of carnivore.

Chapter 5:

The Benefits of the Carnivore Diet

Jordan Peterson is one of our all-time favorite thinkers. While many of his stances are viewed as controversial, we believe that when you take the time to listen to him talk instead of just listening to sound bites or the mainstream media's take on his opinions, you'll find that he's a lot more practical than he's given credit for.

Dr. Peterson has had quite the health journey dealing with a variety of autoimmune conditions, depression, and anxiety. While these conditions plagued him for much of his life, he was surprised to find that they were largely alleviated when he was introduced to the carnivore diet by his daughter Mikhaila's, who also used the diet to manage her debilitating autoimmune conditions.

On the Joe Rogan Experience Podcast, Dr. Peterson was quoted saying of carnivore, "I lost 50 pounds. My appetite has probably fallen by 70%. I don't get blood sugar dysregulation problems. I need way less sleep... my gum disease is gone. Like, what the hell?" Jordan has also pointed out that carnivore has helped alleviate his symptoms of depression, anxiety, psoriasis, and gastric reflux.

Treating autoimmune conditions, anxiety, and depression is no small feat. We're talking about conditions that affect a large number of the population and of which there are few effective treatments. Dr. Peterson and his daughter Mikhaila are not the only individuals who have experienced this either. Visit any social media account or Reddit forum on the topic, and you'll find thousands of others who have experienced similar benefits.

It's true that all of the potential health benefits of the carnivore diet have not been extensively studied in a clinical setting. However, the sheer number of anecdotes from doctors and patients makes it hard to ignore all that this way of eating can provide. But we know that anecdotal evidence isn't always the strongest, so in this chapter, you will often see us looking to keto research to provide scientific support for the benefits we and many others are experiencing on carnivore.

Here are a few of the most notable benefits of a carnivore diet.

Weight Loss

One of the big reasons why carnivore has become so popular is because of its weight loss potential. Carnivore is a variation of a low-carb diet, and it is no secret that low-carb diets are incredibly effective when it comes to weight loss.

It's a very simple formula. When you restrict your carbohydrate intake, your insulin levels lower. When insulin levels are low, your body burns more fat. Following a low-carb diet actually puts your body in prime fat-burning mode.

Due to some of the upcoming benefits, carnivore also tends to lead to calorie restriction. While research shows us that calories are not the only determining factor of weight loss success, they still play a role, and caloric restriction due to carnivore dieting contributes to the weight loss experienced on the diet.

Reduced Hunger

Chris's friend Jake has always been a snacker. And not just a "snack here and there" type of a snacker – but an all-day, even-if-he-just-finished-a-meal type of a snacker. Ever since he was a kid, Jake had an ever-present hunger that he could never seem to satisfy.

When he was younger, this wasn't as much of a problem. Jake was an athlete growing up, so he was always moving, running, training – and burning calories. As Jake got older, however, his lifestyle changed. He started working a desk job, his daily activity decreased, and he no longer had the time or energy to train as he did when he was a kid. Unfortunately, the one thing that did stay the same was his strong desire to snack. In a relatively short time, Jake's sedentary lifestyle, coupled with his insatiable hunger, led to an extra 20 pounds of weight gain, and despite his best efforts, he just couldn't seem to shake it.

Jake was one of Chris's first friends to try a carnivore diet after Chris introduced him to the concept. While he was a little skeptical at first, he decided to give it a go, not realizing that his relationship with food was about to change drastically. After just a few days on the carnivore diet, Jake found that for the first time in his life, he no longer desired snacks after or between his meals. For someone who had been a chronic snacker their entire life, this was a game changer. He reported feeling significantly less hungry throughout the day, leading to much better appetite control and a reduction in his total daily calorie consumption. Over a few months, Jake lost those stubborn 20 pounds that plagued him for so many years, and he finally felt empowered in his relationship with food.

Reduced hunger is a benefit of carnivore that's particularly interesting to us. It's well established that keto, in general, has a potent ability to reduce hunger through several different mechanisms, such as improved appetite signaling, reductions in hunger hormones, and blood sugar stability[1]. While these mechanisms would also be in play for carnivore, there seems to be something else going on as well.

The carnivore diet is not hyper-palatable, meaning there isn't much flavor. On keto, you'll still find hyper-palatable foods (think of a Cobb salad with all its variety: steak, eggs, greens, blue cheese, nuts, and salad dressing). While this plethora of flavor is certainly enjoyable, it comes at a price: it can stimulate additional hunger.

On a 100% carnivore diet, you're only eating meat. While meat is delicious, it lacks variety and flavor, it's not hyper-palatable, and diets that are not hyper-palatable make it easier to stay full and prevent overeating. Simple as that.

Now, here's the flip side. While this lack of hunger can be beneficial for those trying to restrict calories or control appetite, it can also make it hard to eat enough. Calorie restriction is good, but chronic severe calorie restriction is not, which is why you may need to start tracking calories if you start noticing symptoms like fatigue, lack of strength, and poor recovery from the gym.

Lower Blood Sugar & Insulin

Blood sugar and insulin are incredibly important markers of metabolic health. Unfortunately, over 90% of the adult population in the U.S. is suffering from poor metabolic health, which means more than 90% have less-than-ideal blood sugar and insulin levels.

When blood sugar levels are constantly spiking, we eventually develop what is known as insulin resistance. Insulin resistance prevents the hormone insulin from doing its job of getting sugar out of the blood, resulting in both higher insulin and blood glucose levels. Insulin resistance is prediabetes, and one-third of our adult population here in the U.S. is thought to be suffering from it.

Low-carb diets are a great way to lower blood sugar and insulin levels, and carnivore is no exception. Like weight loss, the formula here is easy: fewer carbs = lower blood sugar = lower insulin. Carnivore is essentially a zero-carb diet, which is why we're now hearing carnivore success stories from individuals with type 2 diabetes.

In fact, a study published by Harvard University looking at over 2,000 participants following a carnivore diet reported that 100% of diabetics in the study came off of injectable medications, 92% came off insulin completely, and 84% came off of all oral diabetes medications[2]. Those are pretty impressive results, especially coming from an organization that less than a year later published low-quality data saying red meat consumption is associated with an increased risk of type 2 diabetes (eye roll).

Those familiar with a keto diet may have concerns about the high protein nature of carnivore and its impact on blood sugar due to the phenomenon known as gluconeogenesis, a process that converts protein into glucose. It's important to note that this process is demand-driven and not supply-driven, meaning the body does not ramp up gluconeogenesis just because we eat more protein. Even on a keto diet, we don't believe you should fear protein.

Ketosis

Due to the low-carb, high-protein, and high-fat nature of the carnivore diet, this way of eating can shift your body into a state of ketosis. As your body senses that there aren't enough carbohydrates coming in to make sufficient glucose, it will turn its metabolic levers to favor fat-burning. As your body ramps up its fat-burning mechanisms, it will begin to produce ketones to take the place of glucose, and voila – you're in a state of ketosis.

The ketogenic diet has become increasingly popular in the last decade or so, which means that we have a fair amount of research backing the benefits of ketosis. While a carnivore diet isn't synonymous with a ketogenic diet, if you're following a carnivore diet correctly, it should increase your ketone production.

Some of the most well-researched benefits of ketosis and the keto diet include:[3,4,5,6]

- Appetite regulation
- Weight loss
- Improved lipid profiles (reduced LDL cholesterol, increased HDL cholesterol)
- Improved blood sugar control
- Reduced inflammation
- Improved outcomes in neurological disease
- Improved gut microbiota

At its core, the keto diet is highly anti-inflammatory, which is one of the reasons that we see so many potential benefits when people choose to cut carbs. With carnivore, you get all of the benefits keto has to offer – and then some.

Decreased Inflammation

If you look at nearly any chronic disease, you'll find inflammation playing a role in some form or fashion. The keto diet is already well known for lowering inflammation via reduced production of reactive oxygen species and the ability for ketones to increase our natural antioxidant defenses[7].

Carnivore seems to possess an even more potent ability to reduce inflammation, which has been reported by many. Although carnivore may not have the robust research that keto can claim, many people who try carnivore show significant improvements in inflammatory symptoms and markers. One well-known proponent includes film director Chris Bell, who uses the diet to manage his arthritis. Anecdotally, Chris found that after following carnivore for eight weeks, he measured the lowest c-reactive protein reading (a common inflammatory marker) he's ever registered before – on any diet.

It's worth mentioning that the inflammation-lowering benefits of carnivore aren't well accepted because we've been taught that eating red meat will increase inflammation. However, this claim is not supported by research. In fact, several published articles show just the opposite. For example, one group of researchers had 60 participants replace carbohydrate-rich foods with 200g/d of red meat per day for eight weeks. The results from the study found that the meat group had lower markers of oxidative stress and inflammation, leading the researchers to conclude that increases in red meat intake are unlikely to increase oxidative stress or inflammation and may even offer a protective effect[8].

RESEARCH SPOTLIGHT:

DOES RED MEAT CAUSE INFLAMMATION?

Many people think that consuming red meat will increase inflammation but what does the research say?

Study Design:	60 Subjects were randomized to either maintain their diet or replace carb rich foods with 200g/d of lean red meat for 8 weeks. Calories were the same Common inflammatory marker **C-Reactive Protein** was measured at baseline and after 8 weeks.
Results:	Those eating red meat did not increase c-reactive protein but rather had a trend for lower c-reactive protein levels
Conclusion:	UNPROCESSED red meat does not increase inflammation and many have reported that it decreases it

Citation: Hodgson et al 2012

Hormone Production

As a population, an increasing number of adults are being affected by hormone deficiencies. particularly sex-hormones. This is a big reason why we're seeing an increase in reproductive-related health complications like PCOS, infertility, and low testosterone in males.

High-fat diets tend to lend themselves to improved hormonal production due to the importance of cholesterol and saturated fat in this process. Research shows us that lowering fat intake and increasing fiber intake results in a decrease in testosterone[9]. and that a ketogenic diet can provide a boost in testosterone levels[10]. A carnivore diet may be even better at this due to its focus on red meat, which is loaded with saturated fat and cholesterol. These fats, despite getting a bad reputation, are important for the production of hormones and are one of the reasons why many report better energy and sexual function while on a carnivore diet.

If you recall from Chapter 2, some of the compounds found in plants can also impact hormone levels in a negative way, which is another part of the reason why cutting plants out can provide hormonal balance.

Muscle Growth

The same study mentioned in the section on inflammation, where large amounts of meat were added to the subject's diet, also demonstrated increases in testosterone, decreases in fat mass, and increases in lean body mass, supporting the fact that low-carb, high-fat diets can stimulate muscle growth. Unsurprisingly, increased lean body mass and muscle growth are among the most commonly reported outcomes from people following the carnivore diet.

Improved hormone levels help, but another factor that influences muscle gain with a carnivore diet is an increase in high-quality protein intake. Meat is rich in protein and, in particular, the essential amino acid leucine. Leucine is important for stimulating muscle protein synthesis, which is the anabolic process your body needs in order to increase muscle mass and support muscle recovery. Having a diet rich in high-quality protein gives your muscles the fuel they need to rebuild.

The presence of ketones also plays a role in the muscle benefits of carnivore. Ketones have been shown to be "muscle sparing," meaning they prevent the breakdown of leucine[11]. There's also some evidence suggesting that ketones may be able to stimulate muscle protein synthesis[12].

You can't talk about muscle growth without mentioning the effort required in the gym to make it happen. You can eat all the protein you want, but if you are not properly stimulating your muscles, growth isn't just going to happen. Carnivore helps in this area as well, increasing energy and strength in the gym so you can push your body to adapt to resistance training with muscle growth.

Better Exercise Performance

When we both began our careers in health, it was a known "fact" that carbohydrates were the essential fuel for exercise, especially endurance exercise. It's now becoming widely accepted that low-carb diets can be great for all exercise performance, especially endurance performance[13,14].

One of our favorite low-carb stories is from a friend of Chris named Eric who was already an incredible endurance athlete before learning about the potential of the ketogenic diet. After spending over a year training in a fat-adapted state, Eric went out and set a new marathon PR. The kicker….he did it in a fasted state—no sugar gels every couple of miles like before.

The idea with low-carb dieting and endurance performance is that when we restrict our carbohydrate intake, our bodies are forced to tap into fat for fuel, which we store much more of compared to carbohydrates, allowing us to maintain superior exercise performance for extended periods of time. Additionally, red meat is rich in the amino acid creatine, which is one of the most research-backed compounds for improving muscle strength and endurance[15].

While there's not a lot of research looking directly at the carnivore diet's impact on exercise performance, there are plenty of anecdotal stories reporting improvements. Here is a quote from actor, carnivore advocate, and health coach William Shewfelt:

"The Carnivore Diet, in my experience, has been an absolute performance enhancer. When I transitioned to carnivore—a few things happened. My satiety increased. My strength increased without changing my training. My lean mass went up, and my fat mass went down. I subjectively felt stronger, faster, and a lot more energetic throughout the day. I believe the removal of plant antigens and the increase in protein and nutrients thanks to red meat, eggs, and seafood helped my body repair from the training stimulus better than ever. My training is based on both aerobic endurance and strength. Aerobically, I'm in the best shape of my life thanks to ketones. Strength-wise, I'm stronger than ever. Red meat is the poor man's steroids."

This quote summarizes much of what we already talked about. The increase in high-quality protein and boost in hormone production on carnivore, as well as the ability to tap into stored fat and produce ketones on the diet, is a big reason why so many people are reporting improved exercise performance from going all meat.

Better Exercise Recovery

When Chris first started following a ketogenic diet, he was blown away by the wide array of benefits he experienced. Particularly when it came to sports performance; that said, during his early days on the diet (when his food wasn't quite optimized yet), he found that his recovery from training was a bit impaired. Although he could push through his workouts, his muscles would take a while to recuperate, and he found it difficult to string together a few days of hard training in a row.

Through experimentation, Chris discovered that increasing his protein and calorie intake helped alleviate the majority of his recovery woes. While this was a step in the right direction, once Chris went full carnivore, he found that the protein density of his diet took his exercise performance and recovery to a whole new level. Simply put, his need for rest became days were few and far between.

A higher protein intake and subsequent stimulation of protein synthesis are definitely at the top of the list for contributing to better muscle repair following exercise. However, the anti-inflammatory nature of carnivore also plays a role since acute exercise-induced inflammation is a big reason that muscle soreness exists in the first place.

The nutrient density of meat, which we'll cover in the coming chapters, is also worth highlighting here. When your body is receiving ample key micronutrients, the processes that support muscle growth and recovery are going to be optimized.

Improved Mood

Another underappreciated benefit of the carnivore diet is the impact it can have on our mood. Amber O'hearn, one of the trailblazers for using carnivore to balance mood, credits carnivore with resolving her bipolar depression and suicidal thoughts. Both of which medication was unable to alleviate. Combine this with what Dr. Peterson experienced, and you have two of the thousands of incredible stories that exist about the mood-boosting potential of carnivore.

But It's not just anecdotes that support this idea. A very interesting review published in 2021 in the Journal of Food Science and Nutrition examined 20 studies, including over 170,000 participants, and found that eating more red meat was associated with better mood[16]. In fact, the study found that the more meat people ate, the lower their depression and anxiety were. Meanwhile, vegan and vegetarian diets were linked with an increased likelihood of depression and psychiatric disorders. This was not the first study to find a link between a lack of meat consumption and an increased risk of depression either[17].

One of the reasons that we see plant-based diets driving mood disorders is the nutrient component of these diets. When you cut out meat, you also severely reduce your intake of vitamin B12, zinc, creatine, and taurine – all nutrients that are important for mood.

Another mechanism for the mood-boosting effects of carnivore is the metabolic health improvements this diet can provide. Thanks to the work of experts like Dr. Christopher Palmer, we are now finding that metabolic health and mental health are deeply associated with one another; thus, improving metabolic health is a great strategy for improving mental health.

It's also worth mentioning that ketosis has strong mood-boosting capabilities due to many factors, such as improving neurotransmitter production and decreasing inflammation in the brain

Cognitive Function

It is not uncommon to hear carnivore dieters talking raging about the cognitive benefits of the diet. Similar to keto, this is due to several factors.

Blood sugar control and increases in energy tell at least part of the story here, but it is also well-established that ketosis can boost brain function due to the unique utilization of ketones by the brain. Interestingly, research has shown that ketones are the preferred fuel source of the brain, demonstrated by the fact that when both glucose and ketones are present, the brain will decrease glucose utilization and opt for ketones as its fuel source[18]. This is thought to be driven by the fact that ketones provide more energy to this organ (the brain) that has the highest energy demand in the body, and it does so while producing fewer inflammatory molecules and boosting anti-oxidant production in the brain. All factors that can boost brain function.

The Gut-Brain Axis

Since we are talking about the role of carnivore in mood and brain function, we have to point out that part of the reason for these benefits is the impact carnivore has on the gut, thanks to the gut-brain axis.

The gut-brain axis is an intricate communication network that links the central nervous system, which includes the brain and spinal cord, with the enteric nervous system of the gastrointestinal tract and the gut microbiome. This bi-directional pathway utilizes neural, hormonal, and immunological signals to maintain communication and a relationship between these two seemingly separate systems of the body.

The most notable impact of this relationship is seen in neurotransmitters. Neurotransmitters, which include serotonin, dopamine, acetylcholine, norepinephrine, and gamma-aminobutyric acid (GABA), are chemical messengers that the body transmits from one nerve cell to other cells, influencing everything from muscle contractions to mood, thoughts, sleep, and even heart rate.

Interestingly, while it is assumed that neurotransmitter production only has to do with the brain, the gut is a significant player. In fact, 90% of the neurotransmitter serotonin, which is crucial for mood regulation, is produced in the gut, meaning its production is related to the function of the digestive system and the gut microbiome. The gut microbiome also influences the production of other neurotransmitters, including GABA, dopamine, and norepinephrine, all of which play roles in mood and cognitive function.

So, what impact does gut health actually have on mood and cognitive function?

Research has shown that a healthy gut microbiome is related to positive mood and cognitive performance, while a poor microbiome is related to mood disorders. An imbalanced gut microbiome can lead to increased intestinal permeability ("leaky gut"), allowing endotoxins to enter circulation and trigger inflammation, further contributing to mood disorders.

The hypothalamic-pituitary-adrenal (HPA) axis, a critical part of our stress response system, is also influenced by signals from the gut. A compromised gut can lead to an exaggerated stress response or stress-related pathologies.

Emerging research suggests that the gut-brain axis may also influence memory, decision-making, and other cognitive functions through various mechanisms, including inflammation, hormonal pathways, and direct neural communication.

Productivity

Admittedly, this is a total anecdote with little to no scientific evidence supporting it, but we truly believe that an underappreciated benefit of carnivore is the boost in productivity you can experience.

Of course, some of this boost in productivity is due to the mood, cognitive, and energy-boosting effects of being in ketosis. However, we think the real magic is in the lack of hunger and simplicity of the diet. As we mentioned in the last chapter, Chris first noticed this benefit when he was writing his first book, Keto Answers. Whenever he goes into a very mentally taxing project, he does his best to optimize his lifestyle to accommodate for the focus and clarity he needs to complete the project. When he was writing Keto Answers, he decided to give carnivore a try and was blown away by what he experienced.

Since carnivore is so simple, the amount of time and energy he had to spend on shopping and prepping his food was drastically reduced. Even more, he didn't think about food much, which allowed him to maintain a focused workflow for hours at a time. He allowed this to manifest itself into OMAD (one meal a day) carnivore. While this may not have been the best overall approach for, say, muscle growth or exercise recovery, since his primary focus was optimizing creative output, he leaned into it and now uses the carnivore diet as a tool anytime he really needs to prioritize his work output.

Improved Autoimmune Symptoms

We've experienced a stark rise in autoimmune diagnoses over the last couple of decades. Conditions like Hashimoto's disease, rheumatoid arthritis, lupus, Crohn's Disease, and multiple sclerosis (MS) are all on the rise. While it's likely that much of this increase is a result of better understanding, identification, and diagnosis of autoimmune conditions, there's no doubt that this problem is affecting a lot more people today than it ever has.

Today, more than 100 different autoimmune conditions exist, and over 50 million Americans are dealing with at least one of those conditions – 75% of which are women. Autoimmune conditions can manifest in a variety of ways, including issues we have already discussed, like poor digestive function, acne, poor mental health, and arthritis.

Mikhaela Peterson (now Fuller) was one of the first mainstream anecdotes we heard about the carnivore diet improving autoimmune conditions. Mikhaela suffered from severe autoimmunity since she was a child. She dealt with incredible pain and even had to have her joints replaced when she was just a young girl. Mikhaila reported that carnivore was able to alleviate many of her autoimmune symptoms, including the depression and fatigue that accompanied her condition.

Admittedly, there's not a lot of research on this topic yet, so we have a long way to go. One major line of scientific support we do have on this topic comes from monumental case studies published by Dr. Steven Gundry looking at individuals with autoimmune conditions removing lectins and seeing complete resolution of autoimmune and inflammatory markers in nearly 95% of subjects, and 80% were able to get off of immunosuppressant medications[19].

Regardless of the clinical evidence, the mounting anecdotal evidence is becoming hard to refute. Especially when combined with the mechanisms by which this diet can provide benefits. With around 70-80% of your immune cells being present in the gut, you can imagine how focusing on gut healing may improve autoimmune symptoms and outcomes.

Gut Reset

In our opinion, one of the strongest benefits of a carnivore diet is what it can do for your gut health. Which, if you haven't noticed by now, is also a big reason for all of the other benefits we discussed throughout this chapter.

A carnivorous diet is essentially an elimination diet because you're cutting out all foods that aren't meat. Due to the antinutrients and other compounds found in plant foods that can cause digestive flare-ups, carnivore allows for a type of gut reset that can be just what the doctor ordered if you have digestive issues.

As we'll get into in the coming chapters, it's not just the removal of plant toxins that allows carnivore to improve gut health. Meat also contains specific nutrients that can help improve the structure and integrity of your gut lining, which, as mentioned in Chapter 1, is huge for optimizing gut health.

Another significant benefit of carnivore for gut healing is the temporary, complete removal of carbohydrates from your diet. Gram-negative bacteria love to feed off of sugar, it's what they thrive on. When you eliminate carbs from your diet, you essentially starve unhealthy bacteria and prevent them from propagating. Thus, the carnivore diet makes your gut an uninhabitable home for unhealthy bacteria.

While research is still limited on carnivore for gut health, a small study published in 2020 found that five out of six subjects improved SIBO with a carnivore diet[20]. With what we've seen so far, we feel confident that there will be plenty of future studies examining the benefits of carnivore for gut health, and look forward to sharing those studies as they're published.

What's the Deal with #meatheals?

After reading about all of these potential benefits of the carnivore diet, you may be thinking that carnivore is some type of panacea. Especially since carnivore has blown up and people are now using the hashtag #meatheals on social media. While we do believe that meat does have the ability to heal and can provide a myriad of benefits, especially for people suffering from autoimmunity and poor gut health, we want to point out that some of the benefits of carnivore are a result of what you're cutting out of your diet. Remember what Dr. Ede said: do not mistake a diet for something because of something it is not.

When the Inuit people, who were previously eating primarily meat, were first introduced to carbohydrates, researchers demonstrated increases in hypertension and diabetes[21]. This wasn't necessarily because the meat they were eating was keeping these diseases at bay; it was because they were not eating carbohydrates.

This isn't to take away from the power of carnivore but rather to point out that some of the benefits highlighted in this chapter are a result of the removal of plant foods and other junk ingredients that typically make up the Standard American Diet.

Chapter 6:

Is the Carnivore Diet Safe?

If you're anything like us, then we're sure the first time you heard about carnivore, you were a bit skeptical. It does go against basically everything we've ever been told about nutrition and health. Trust us, we get it.

From the very first nutrition class we ever took, we had both been taught to fear meat and fat. We still remember going to grocery stores, looking at food labels, and being appalled at how much fat and cholesterol were in so many of the foods. We both remember thinking that this has to be the reason why our society is so sick.

Boy, were we wrong.

As we have both continued our exploration of nutrition and its role in chronic disease, we have found that the evidence supporting meat and fat, especially cholesterol and saturated fat, being the cause of chronic disease is weak. In fact, the more you look at the research, the more you realize how important these nutrients are to optimal health.

All of this forced our curious minds to delve deeper into the "why" behind the societal fear of meat and fat, which led us both to discover that the "research" saying meat and fat are bad for you is complete and utter bullshit.

Let's start here.

Why Do People Think Meat is Unhealthy?

There are entire books dedicated to answering this question; one of the best is The Big Fat Surprise by Nina Teicholz. We'll try to summarize as best as possible.

In the mid-1900s, a perfect recipe for scrutinizing saturated fat and meat was created. All the recipe called for was a spoonful of political interest, a pinch of cherry-picked data, and a splash of flawed nutrition science. One of the key chefs was a researcher by the name of Ancel Keys.

Ancel Keys was an American physiologist and nutritionist who conducted research on the relationship between diet and health. He's most famous for developing the "diet-heart hypothesis," which posits that a diet high in saturated fat leads to an increased risk of heart disease.

The problem is that the data used to support Ancel's hypothesis turned out to be cherry-picked and influenced by political interests. One of Keys' famous studies, "The Seven Countries Study" reported that countries with the lowest rates of heart disease ate the least amount of saturated fat. The problem is Keys intentionally left France and Switzerland out of his report because the data from those countries found the opposite, skewing his results.

Another major study from Ancel was "The Minnesota Coronary Experiment," which was conducted in the 1960s. The purpose of this study was to test the diet-heart hypothesis in 9,000 participants, splitting them up into either high or low-saturated fat diets. This study found NO DIFFERENCE in heart disease outcomes between the two groups. The problem? The data from this study wasn't published until several *decades* later.

You may be wondering, how did this research get taken to "heart" then? To understand, you have to have a bit of context behind what else was happening during the time this research was coming out.

In 1955, President Dwight D. Eisenhower had a heart attack while serving in office. As you might expect, this was a shocking event. It was so shocking that it led to a robust increase in awareness and fear of heart disease amongst the American population. During this time, governing health and nutrition bodies were clamoring for advice to give to the fearful public. Since the diet-heart hypothesis was popular at the time, it was adopted, leading to a widespread fear of saturated fat and, thus, red meat in general. A fear that still plagues our society today.

What's crazy is that despite more and more people realizing the flaws in the justification for fear of saturated fat, there's still research like this being published year after year:

Dietary fat intake and risk of cardiovascular disease and all-cause mortality in a population at high risk of cardiovascular disease 🆓

PREDIMED Study Investigators

The American Journal of Clinical Nutrition, Volume 102, Issue 6, December 2015, Pages 1563–1573, https://doi.org/10.3945/ajcn.115.116046

Published: 11 November 2015   **Article history** ▾

The problem with studies like this and the studies Ancel Keys was publishing is that they're weak and can only demonstrate correlation and not causation.

In studies like these, individuals are selected and analyzed for cardiovascular disease risk and then questioned about their diets. The answers to these questions are used to formulate the conclusion of the studies. If a significant number of people with high CVD risk answer that they're eating hamburgers, it's assumed that meat and fat, especially saturated fat, is the cause of this increased risk of CVD.

We cannot assume that because someone diagnosed with heart disease is eating a lot of saturated fat, that fat is the cause of the disease. Especially if the subjects were not even asked if they were also eating carbohydrates. Hint, Hint. What about the bun on that hamburger? Or maybe the high fructose corn syrup ketchup? Or the side of fries fried in seed oils? Or the 32 oz. soda?

Interestingly, in that same study, it was found that saturated fats from pastries and processed foods were associated with an even higher risk of CVD, which demonstrates that carbohydrates and sugars were likely contributing to the damage. Conveniently, many anti-meat proponents left these results out.

While it was helpful that this study looked at sugar and processed carbs, it failed to look at how many total carbs the subjects with the highest saturated fat intake were also eating. Knowing the trends of human nutrition, we would venture to say this information would have produced significantly different findings.

Unfortunately, studies like this get misconstrued and turned into news headlines with titles like "Saturated Fat Increases the Risk of Heart Disease," which then scare people away from fat and meat.

The take-home message here is that anti-meat propaganda has been built on the back of epidemiological nutrition studies – which are incredibly weak sources of information. These studies look at correlating factors and shed very little light on the true cause of health issues. But even if these studies were highly valuable, when you take a look at the data (in its entirety), you'll actually find that there is little to no association between saturated fat intake and all-cause mortality, coronary heart disease, ischaemic stroke, or type 2 diabetes in healthy adults[1,2].

What we do have, on the other hand, is a great deal of research on keto for cardiovascular health, demonstrating that low-carb, high-fat diets can improve many cardiovascular disease risk factors[3,4,5,6]. Even better is a study looking at 112,000 men and 184,000 women followed for an 11-year period. This study found that red meat was actually *inversely* associated with CVD mortality, meaning that the individuals who ate more red meat had a lower risk of CVD[7]!

But it's not just cardiovascular disease that makes people fearful of meat (and, therefore, a carnivore diet). It turns out there are a lot of similar narratives on other detrimental health impacts of meat, which is a big reason why more and more people are trying vegetarian diets (2 thumbs down). Let's go over a few others.

Digestive Health

One of the big reasons why the carnivore diet has not been widely accepted for digestive health is because of the misconception that meat is bad for your digestive health and fiber is good for it.

In Chapter 2, we did a breakdown of why fiber isn't all it's cracked up to be and even highlighted some research showing how the removal of fiber from the diets of those suffering from various digestive complications, including constipation, led to better digestive outcomes.

No matter how much evidence is presented, many people still believe that fiber is essential under all circumstances. This is largely based on the idea that we need to have a diverse gut microbiome and that fiber will help us get there. While it is true that healthy microbial diversity in the gut can be a good thing, there is no evidence that says fiber is the only way to achieve that. In fact, research looking at low-fiber ketogenic diets has shown that despite the lack of fiber intake, this way of eating doesn't decrease diversity scores[8].

Another prevailing story around fiber is that it is critical for the production of butyrate. Butyrate is a short-chain fatty acid that helps to maintain gut health and ensures the integrity of our intestinal lining. Interestingly, it appears that the amino acid lysine, which is found in meat, can also be converted to butyrate and offer intestinal protection[9]. Again, meat is providing what we need.

This is not the only way a carnivore diet can feed beneficial gut bacteria, though. Molecules produced through the fermentation of protein and the breakdown of fat for fuel can also feed the intestinal cells. Specifically, the fermentation of protein produces isobutyrate, which can be used by the gut cells and also has many other similar actions as butyrate. The ketone bodies acetoacetate and beta-hydroxybutyrate can also serve as a source of energy for gut cells.

It's not just the lack of fiber that has everyone tripped up at carnivore for gut health, though. Over the last few years, there have been a lot of new studies coming out that seem to support the idea that red meat can increase the risk of colorectal cancer. Obviously not ideal for a healthy gut. The issue is that these studies are those weak epidemiological studies we have talked about throughout the book, and they just don't hold up to what happens in real life. Regardless, it turns out that when you account for other lifestyle factors like drinking, smoking, and stress, the association between red meat and colon cancer is nearly non-existent.

From what we have seen in the research, there is no reason to think that eating a diet rich in red meat is going to hurt your digestive health. In fact, as we will cover in the next chapter, the combination of cutting out plant compounds and replacing them with gut health-promoting nutrients found in meat is actually a recipe for improved gut health.

Type 2 Diabetes

The prevailing narrative in mainstream medicine is that red meat is a main driver of type 2 diabetes. The story here is similar to what we just covered for cardiovascular disease—decades of weak research published by anti-meat crusaders with industry-funded biases.

In late 2023, Harvard's Walter Willett published a paper announcing that red and processed meat are "strongly associated" with increased risk of type 2 diabetes, citing that participants in the study who ate the most red meat had "a 62% higher risk of developing type 2 diabetes compared to those who ate the least.[10]"

This paper made national headlines and moved Harvard into its 3+ decade of having an antimeat stance. When you take a deeper dive into Walter Willett's backstory, you find that he has a lot of incentive to be against meat, including his involvement in a vegan-promoting church and the multiple six-figure donations his department has received from the food industry[11]. He was also a colleague of Ancel Keys and was heavily influenced by his work (or, should we say, biases).

Just like cardiovascular disease, there is ample epidemiological evidence showing a relationship between red meat consumption and increased rates of type 2 diabetes—all studies showing similar jaw-dropping statistics as Willett's headlining 2023 paper. Again, epidemiological research fails to take into account the nuance of diet, and most of the reported "red meat" intake in these studies includes fast food hamburgers, hot dogs, pizza toppings, and other highly processed foods that combine red meat with refined carbohydrates, sugar, and trans fats. Of course, consuming a lot of these would increase chronic disease risk, especially type 2 diabetes.

Interestingly, despite the epidemiological-like evidence, if you look at nutrition trends, there has actually been a decline in red meat consumption over the years, and it has coincided with a dramatic increase in diabetes cases, hinting at red meat not being the issue.

Looking past weak epidemiological research at higher quality research is where you get a true look at the science. A review published back in 2022 looking at 21 different randomized controlled trials found that compared to reduced and no red meat diets, eating red meat did not increase insulin resistance, fasting glucose, fasting insulin, HbA1c, or even pancreatic beta-cell function[12]—all the biggest risk factors for type 2 diabetes.

It sounds to me like the mainstream narrative against red meat is being paid for. What do you think?

Cancer

We've all seen the headlines accusing meat of being a cause of cancer, a disease that scares the crap out of us! As it turns out, this story is the same as what we see with heart disease and diabetes: plenty of correlation but no support for causation.

While epidemiological research does exist, when you take a closer look at the data, you find that there's much more than what's being presented in the mainstream narrative.

One of the more recent publications that made a big splash was a paper published in the Lancet titled "Carcinogenicity of consumption of red and processed meat." This study made a lot of headlines because it included the work of 22 scientists from 10 different countries[13]. The conclusion interpreted by many was that red meat consumption was associated with a greater risk of colorectal cancer. Sparking many alarming headlines like:

> Lancet Oncol. 2015 Dec;16(16):1599-600. doi: 10.1016/S1470-2045(15)00444-1. Epub 2015 Oct 29.

Carcinogenicity of consumption of red and processed meat

Véronique Bouvard [1], Dana Loomis [1], Kathryn Z Guyton [1], Yann Grosse [1], Fatiha El Ghissassi [1], Lamia Benbrahim-Tallaa [1], Neela Guha [1], Heidi Mattock [1], Kurt Straif [1]; International Agency for Research on Cancer Monograph Working Group

Collaborators, Affiliations + expand

PMID: 26514947   DOI: 10.1016/S1470-2045(15)00444-1

When you take a deeper look at the study, however, a lot of holes present themselves. For instance, besides the study being epidemiological, meaning it can't show causation, and relying on self-reported dietary intake, which is often inaccurate, the study also failed to differentiate between processed and unprocessed red meat or to account for other lifestyle and environmental factors like drinking, smoking, sleep, exercise, and more.

Again, this type of research is not sufficient for telling us if something is causing a disease or not. Simply put, there are too many other factors at play. The truth is that the evidence that meat causes cancer is weak. Even weaker, in fact, than what we see for cardiovascular disease.

Kidney Damage

Kidney health is also a common concern with carnivore due to the high protein nature of the diet and the assumption that protein is bad for your kidneys. This is also a myth.

According to a review published in the American Journal of Kidney Diseases, "there is no conclusive evidence that high-protein intake negatively affects kidney function in healthy individuals[14]." Additionally, a meta-analysis of several studies found that high-protein diets did not increase the risk of kidney disease in healthy individuals[15].

It's important to note that the above research is on healthy subjects. Individuals with pre-existing kidney disease or reduced kidney function may need to be more mindful of their protein intake, but this is something to take up with your doctor.

So, You're Saying Carnivore is Safe?

All of this information is meant to show you that if you're worried about carnivore because of what you've been told about meat, it may be time to upgrade your thinking.

It's true that we still lack randomized controlled trials looking at the safety of a carnivore diet, but that's only a consequence of the fact that consuming a meat-based diet is still a relatively new concept in modern times.

That said, there are plenty of anecdotes that support the safety of carnivore, like the story of Mr. Vilhjalmur Stefansson, for example.

Stefansson was an Arctic explorer who lived with the Inuit in the early 1900s. He adopted the Inuit diet of fish, wild game, and water, with the occasional seasonal berries. Following this expedition, he and a fellow explorer, Karsen Anderson, ate nothing but meat and water for an entire year under the medical supervision of Bellevue Hospital in New York

City[16]. At the end of the study, both men were reported to be in good physical shape; their teeth showed no signs of deterioration, and they hadn't lost any physical or mental vigor. Further, and in the interest of gut health: "Bowel elimination was undisturbed... The stools were smaller than usual, well-formed, and had an inoffensive, slightly pungent odor. No flatus was noted... The men were not troubled by constipation more than when eating mixed diets. The diet was small in bulk and well absorbed." There was also no clinical evidence of any vitamin deficiencies.

Of course, this old study of two men is far from enough evidence to say this way of eating is safe. However, I think we can make a strong case for its safety if we acknowledge the following facts:

- Animal foods have been a part of the human diet throughout all of history
- Certain civilizations have thrived on eating just meat
- Thousands of people have already used the carnivore diet and have seen incredible improvements in their overall health.

What About the Environmental Impact?

For many people, it's not just the health concerns that make them shy away from eating meat – the environmental impact is another nagging factor.

The truth is that the environmental claims against meat have been drastically overblown, and animal agriculture is not as harmful to our environment as it's often portrayed. In fact, when it is done the right way, it can actually be critically beneficial to our environment, which is why many environmental scientists have deemed regenerative animal agriculture the only path forward.

A popular statistic often cited to frame cattle farming as being environmentally unfriendly comes from the UN Food and Agriculture Association. Their report claimed that cows produce more greenhouse gasses than all of the world's transportation combined, 18%. However, it has since come out that the numbers in this report have been skewed based on biased calculations. In fact, one author from the report has since said that these were "unfair" comparisons and that cows contribute less than 3% of greenhouse gasses.

The truth is that if farming practices are done correctly, cows can serve to be beneficial to the environment. In fact, research shows that grazing cows can help remove carbon from our atmosphere[17] and reduce the natural emissions of nitrous oxide from the land[18]. If you break down the numbers, this actually means that when cows are fed and housed correctly, they can be considered "carbon negative."

Regenerative Agriculture

White Oak Pastures is a regenerative farm that started transitioning away from industrial agriculture techniques in 1995 and is now completely holistically managed. White Oak has published some incredible findings regarding the impact of their farming practices and has found that when managed correctly, cattle can produce a net negative carbon output.

Water use by cows is another environmental concern that you may hear regarding red meat – yet another misconception. If cows are fed how they should be, grazing on the land, then water use is not a problem. In fact, it's feed production that requires the most water use when it comes to raising cattle. Regardless, many of the statistics that look at water use from cattle farming fail to decipher the difference between natural rainfall and irrigation, which leads to water use estimations for cattle being very high and doesn't paint a truthful picture. Research that looks at the water use of non-feedlot animals finds that the amount of non-rainfall water used by cattle is a substantially lower number.

The key theme here is that the environmental impact of animals comes down to how the animals are farmed. It's true that feedlots do not leave the best environmental footprint, but cows that are grazing on the land, living how they're supposed to live, are actually essential to the health of our environment. We highly recommend reading the book Sacred Cow by Robb Wolf and Diana Rodgers to learn more about this topic.

Regenerative Animal Ag & Carbon Emissions

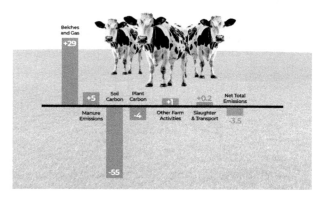

Source: White Oak Pastures

Potential Dangers of Carnivore

We hope by now you can see that the majority of the concerns about the safety of a carnivore diet are not justified or supported by research. However, there are a few potential risks that we think are worth mentioning.

Eating Disorders

Carnivore can be a very restrictive diet, which is why this way of eating may not be best for someone with a history of disordered eating or who currently struggles with their relationship with food. For these individuals, it would be advised only to try something like carnivore with a trained practitioner.

Cooking Your Meat

While we debunked the myths about meat and cancer, it's important to point out that how we cook meat may be important as it relates to cancer risk. Frying meat at super high temperatures for too long and with seed oils may be carcinogenic and should likely be avoided.

When meat is cooked at high temperatures, the amino acids, creatine, and sugars can react with one another to produce heterocyclic amines and (HCAs)[19], which are substances that are thought to be carcinogenic. Similarly, when juices and fat from meat drip into an open flame, like on a grill, for instance, it can create smoke that contains substances known as polycyclic aromatic hydrocarbons (PAHs), which are another potentially carcinogenic toxin.

It's important to note that the National Cancer Institute has only labeled HCA and PAHs as "possible human carcinogens," meaning the evidence is limited. Regardless, the potential risk of various forms of cancer may make it worthwhile to use gentler cooking methods like baking, sous vide, and slow cooking. Research has also shown that the addition of herbs, spices, and marinades can counteract HCA and PAH issues[20,21]. This may not be the best fit for those with severe forms of autoimmunity in need of a more strict carnivore diet, but for the less strict use cases, using these seasonings can be helpful.

Fat Digestion Complications

While there is no reason for most people to fear fat, for individuals with disorders related to fat digestion, there may be reason to pay attention to this aspect of nutrition.

A common "disorder" is found in people who have had their gallbladder removed. The gallbladder stores and releases bile to aid in the digestion of fat. While the liver will also produce bile, individuals who have had their gallbladder removed may struggle to digest a lot of fat. Similarly, individuals with bile duct obstructions may also struggle with fat digestion.

Pancreatic insufficiency is another health complication that can impact fat digestion. The pancreas produces enzymes for the digestion of all the macros, including fat. With conditions like cystic fibrosis or chronic pancreatitis, the pancreas may not secrete enough of the fat digestion enzyme lipase, which is crucial for fat digestion.

Liver disorders can also impair fat digestion. As mentioned, the liver also produces bile, and with conditions like hepatitis, cirrhosis, or fatty liver disease, the production and/or flow of this bile can be impaired.

It's important to point out that if you are dealing with any of these issues, it may not mean that you can't follow a carnivore diet; it might just mean that you will need a little more tailoring of the diet and potentially some medical oversight. Opting for leaner cuts of meats and implementing supplements like ox bile or pancreatic enzymes can help.

Chapter 7:

The Carnivore Diet for Gut Health

Do you remember Megan from the introduction of the book? Megan was Chris's friend who had experienced various forms of digestive distress throughout her life, ultimately resulting in a feeling of helplessness at how much of her life she was losing to these issues. The good news for Megan was that because she had struggled for so long, she was willing to do whatever it took to improve her digestive health and get her life back.

One night, Megan and I were out to dinner with some friends, and Megan mentioned some of the problems she was experiencing. The topic came up naturally because ordering a meal at a restaurant had become quite the task for Megan. She would first need to ensure that the restaurant had gluten-free options because she knew all too well that too much gluten was enough to send her symptoms spiraling out of control. She would then have to ask her server several questions to ensure that the food she ordered didn't contain any of the food allergies and intolerances she had developed, like dairy and eggs. Safe to say, Megan did not enjoy dining out with friends very much and was often embarrassed by her situation.

Knowing my background in nutrition, Megan started asking me questions about what she was experiencing to see if I had any advice. To ensure that I was making the right recommendations, I began asking her more questions about her overall health, which, in turn, led her to realize that many of the other health complications she was experiencing, like acne and anxiety, were also related to her gut issues.

I asked Megan if she had ever tried an elimination diet, to which she responded, "I've tried several juice cleanses, but nothing has helped." No surprise there. As you know by now, drinking a bunch of sugary plant-based juices is unlikely to solve a gut problem. In fact, it's more likely to make it worse.

Megan also mentioned that she had recently tried a vegetarian-based diet several times. While she felt like it helped her initially, in the long run, she felt tired and unmotivated to go to the gym, and her digestive symptoms didn't get much better, so she ultimately decided to abandon her plant-based diet. Again, no surprise there. Throwing a ton of plants on an already impaired gut may be the furthest thing from an optimal solution.

The fact that Megan had tried going plant-based sparked an idea in my head about carnivore. As we'll discuss later in this chapter, there are several nutrients found in meat that are incredibly important for the strength and integrity of our gut lining. If Megan had recently been following a plant-based diet, it was likely that she would benefit from focusing on more meat in her diet.

For this reason, I recommended that Megan try a carnivore diet. I told her that since she was struggling with dairy at the moment, she should try focusing solely on eating meat. Primarily red meat.

Of course, Megan had a lot of questions because she, like many others, thought red meat was bad for her health and was told to limit her intake of meat in general due to her digestive complications. After spending some time debunking the myths she was told, Megan was on board to give it a try. I sent Megan a few blog posts I had written on the topic and told her to let me know if she had any questions or needed any help implementing the diet.

About two weeks later, Megan texted me, saying that she had lost eight pounds so far and was no longer bloated every day. Two to three weeks after that, Megan texted me again, saying her acne had finally cleared up and she was feeling more confident and less anxious at work where previously she would become paralyzed with anxiety.

Eight weeks after their initial conversation, Megan called me and said she couldn't believe how great she felt. By this point, she was down about 15 pounds and said she was no longer experiencing any of the digestive issues she previously had, apart from one night when she tore into the bread basket at a steak restaurant with her husband. Megan was incredibly thankful for having come across carnivore and, to this day, primarily follows an animal-based diet.

At the time, Megan wasn't the only person blown away by the success she experienced on the diet. I was, too. Knowing what I know now, I shouldn't have been.

In order to elicit any sort of major health improvement, you've got to have a strategy in place. And when it comes to gut health, we believe carnivore is a really good strategy. The carnivore diet eliminates all major dietary triggers, including the most insulting of foods like grains, refined carbs, and vegetable oils, and replaces them with foods rich in gut-strengthening nutrients. Besides the benefits of removing triggers and eating gut-strength-promoting foods, carnivore also keeps things simple. There's not a lot of wiggle room for justifications that you'll find with other diets. On carnivore, you can more easily determine if a food is a "yes" or a "no," which makes this way of eating a much easier prescription to follow.

The carnivore diet is not magic, though. Let's dive into the two primary ways carnivore can help strengthen the gut and alleviate digestive complications.

Reason #1: Gut Structure and Integrity

We've discussed how plants are often inferior to meat as far as nutrient density and bioavailability go, but we've only briefly touched on the robust benefits of animal-based foods. The truth is that meat and animal foods are the most nutrient-dense foods for humans. These foods contain all of the essential amino acids, vitamins, and minerals our bodies need to survive and thrive. And the best part is, they're also in a form that's better absorbed (more bioavailable) by humans.

The importance of the bioavailability of these nutrients is highly relevant when we talk about gut health. For starters, vitamin D[1], vitamin A[2], and zinc deficiencies[3] have all been associated with leaky gut and an increased risk of inflammation. If you recall from Chapter 3, each of these nutrients is most bioavailable in animal foods.

Additionally, there are plenty of other nutrients found in animal foods that can support gut health and promote gut repair, such as:
- Vitamin A
- Vitamin D
- Vitamin B12
- Zinc
- DHA & EPA (omega-3 fats)

- Collagen
- Glutamine
- Tryptophan

These nutrients are important to gut health because they play a role in the structure and integrity of our gut. If we want to reset and restore our gut health, we have to improve the structural integrity of our gut lining and combat leaky gut.

Let's go over each of the nutrients essential to gut health, strength, and integrity:

Vitamin A

Vitamin A is a fat-soluble vitamin required for the production and maintenance of the intestinal lining. Vitamin A also supports the growth and differentiation of immune cells, such as T-cells and B-cells, which play a crucial role in maintaining gut immunity. In addition, vitamin A helps to regulate the production of mucus in the gut, which, if you remember, aids in the digestion and absorption of nutrients. A deficiency in vitamin A can lead to various gastrointestinal disorders, including diarrhea, inflammatory bowel disease, and malabsorption syndromes.

Vitamin D

Vitamin D is another fat-soluble vitamin most recognized for its role in the absorption and utilization of calcium, which is required for the formation and maintenance of healthy bones. However, vitamin D is also essential for gut health. Vitamin D receptors are present in the cells lining the intestinal tract, and they're involved in regulating the immune system's response to pathogens and inflammation. Vitamin D also supports the growth and differentiation of T-cells and B-cells, which again play a crucial role in maintaining gut immunity. In addition, vitamin D helps to maintain the integrity of the intestinal barrier, which prevents the entry of harmful substances into the bloodstream. A deficiency in vitamin D can lead to various gastrointestinal disorders, including inflammatory bowel disease, irritable bowel syndrome, and colorectal cancer.

Vitamin B12

Vitamin B12 is an essential vitamin that plays a vital role in the production of red blood cells and the proper functioning of the nervous system, which includes the enteric nervous system that regulates gut motility and function. Vitamin B12 also plays a crucial role in maintaining the intestinal lining, which is why a deficiency in vitamin B12 can lead to several gastrointestinal problems, including tongue inflammation, mouth ulcers, constipation, and diarrhea.

Zinc

Zinc is an essential nutrient required for the growth and maintenance of the cells lining the intestinal tract. This mineral is also involved in the production of antibodies and cytokines, which help to fight off infections and reduce inflammation in the gut. Additionally, zinc is required for the proper functioning of digestive enzymes, which aid in the breakdown and absorption of nutrients. A zinc deficiency can lead to various gastrointestinal disorders, including diarrhea, malabsorption syndromes, and impaired immune function.

DHA & EPA

Eicosapentaenoic acid (EPA) and docosahexaenoic acid (DHA) are omega-3 fatty acids that play a crucial role in reducing inflammation in the gut by regulating the production of pro-inflammatory cytokines. They also support the growth and maintenance of the intestinal lining and help regulate the gut microbiome by promoting the growth of beneficial bacteria and reducing the growth of harmful bacteria. In addition, EPA and DHA have been shown to improve symptoms of inflammatory bowel disease, including ulcerative colitis and Crohn's disease.

Collagen

Collagen is the most abundant protein in the body and is found in the skin, bones, and connective tissues. In the gut, collagen is a major component of the extracellular matrix, which provides structural support to the intestinal lining to maintain the integrity of the intestinal barrier. Collagen also supports the growth and differentiation of intestinal epithelial cells, which play a crucial role in nutrient absorption and immune function. In addition, collagen supplementation has been shown to improve symptoms of gastrointestinal disorders, including leaky gut syndrome, irritable bowel syndrome, and inflammatory bowel disease.

Glutamine

Glutamine is the most abundant amino acid in the bloodstream and is particularly important for the health of the intestinal lining. Glutamine is required for the growth and maintenance of the cells lining the intestinal tract and also supports the growth and differentiation of those T and B immune cells that are important for gut immunity. Glutamine is also involved in the production of mucus in the gut and has been shown to be particularly beneficial for individuals with gastrointestinal disorders, including inflammatory bowel disease, leaky gut syndrome, and chemotherapy-induced mucositis.

Tryptophan

Tryptophan is an essential amino acid that's a precursor for the production of serotonin, a neurotransmitter that plays a crucial role in regulating mood, appetite, and gastrointestinal function. Serotonin is produced in the enterochromaffin cells of the gut lining and has been shown to impact gut motility and function significantly. Tryptophan is also a precursor for the production of melatonin. This hormone regulates the sleep-wake cycle, has been shown to have antioxidant and anti-inflammatory properties, and is essential for optimal digestive function. Additionally, tryptophan regulates the immune system and has been shown to improve gut barrier function and reduce inflammation in the gut. Tryptophan deficiency is linked to various gastrointestinal disorders, including irritable bowel syndrome and inflammatory bowel disease.

The vitamins and minerals listed in this section all play a unique role in the structure and function of our digestive system. Deficiency in these nutrients, which is very common in our society, especially on SAD and plant-based diets, can initiate a cascade of events leading to poor gut health and the subsequent symptoms that dysregulated digestion can produce.

Reason #2: Removal of Plant Toxins and Sensitivities

If you recall the quote from Dr. Ede from earlier in the book, it's not just about what a diet is. It's also about what it is not. A carnivore diet brings a lot to the table, like the key gut health-promoting nutrients found in meat. But part of what makes carnivore work is what it is not, or rather, what you are not getting in your diet when you only eat meat, which is those plant compounds we talked about back in Chapter 2.

Remember, some people tolerate the plant compounds we've discussed in this book with no problem. But for those of you dealing with digestive issues, it is likely that these plant compounds are impairing your gut function and the absorption of nutrients essential to gut health. The evidence we presented in Chapter 2 makes a strong case that it is these plant toxins that are causing or significantly contributing to digestive complications. However, we do not have definitive research that says they are the root cause of digestive issues or autoimmunity or if something else is the root cause, and these plant compounds are wreaking havoc as a result of that root cause. It's likely a combination of with some situations arising from genetics, chronic overconsumption of harmful plant compounds, or medications altering the composition of our gut and creating opportunities for these compounds to inflict damage. Instead of getting hung up on the "chicken or the egg" debate, we feel that given the way the body handles these compounds, if you are dealing with a compromised digestive system and a dysfunctional microbiome, cutting them out makes sense and works by allowing your digestive system to rest and repair itself.

You may ask what evidence we have that removing plant compounds can improve your digestive health. The truth is not a ton. This has not been a field of study that has garnered much attention, and much of the research efforts have been directed at proving the benefit these compounds have on gut health. However, we do have some interesting studies that we can infer from. The study we presented in the section on fiber in Chapter 2 demonstrated how cutting out fiber can alleviate symptoms in those dealing with various digestive issues. We also have those case studies we discussed in Chapter 5, published by Dr. Steven Gundry, which reported that removing lectins in individuals with autoimmune conditions led to 95% of subjects seeing complete resolution of autoimmune and inflammatory markers, and 80% were able to get off of immunosuppressant medications[4].

We also have anecdotal evidence from thousands of people who have experienced robust digestive improvements from the carnivore diet. The science community will tell you that anecdotal evidence doesn't count and that we need rigorous clinical trials to tell us what we need to know about nutrition. The problem, besides the fact that so much nutrition research is paid for by Big Food, is that these studies simply aren't happening. At least not at the scale they need to be to get the evidence that scientists, doctors, and governing health agencies would consider adequate to base recommendations on. What are we supposed to do? Nothing? We believe that what matters most is what happens in real life, and carnivore has improved both our health and countless individuals around us. We don't need a clinical trial to tell us that's a good thing.

The main takeaway from this chapter is that carnivore is not some miracle diet, a misconception that often discredits this way of eating. The methods of action behind the benefits of carnivore are actually pretty simple and reasonable. This diet is essentially an elimination diet that removes specific foods known to cause digestive distress and impair gut function. What differentiates carnivore from other elimination diets, however, is its ability to compound this elimination with nutrients required to rebuild the strength and integrity of your gut lining—a double whammy for digestive restoration.

Chapter 8:

How to Use a Carnivore Diet as an Elimination Diet

If you or someone you know has struggled with gut health and digestive issues and have sought out advice from dietitians or nutritionists, it's likely that you've heard of elimination diets.

Elimination diets, also known as exclusion diets, are dietary protocols that can be used as diagnostic tools to determine which foods are causing allergic reactions or sensitivities leading to various health complications, especially digestive issues. Today, there are several different types of elimination diets ranging from less restrictive protocols like paleo to more restrictive, like the low FODMAP diet and the autoimmune protocol (AIP) diet.

Despite the popularity of elimination diets today, they have actually been around in some form or fashion for centuries. Elimination diets especially rose in popularity in the early 1900s when researchers discovered that certain foods could trigger allergic reactions and cause symptoms such as hives, swelling, and difficulty breathing. This led to the development of the first elimination protocols, which were designed to identify and eliminate allergenic foods from a person's diet.

Elimination diets continued to gain popularity in the 1920s and 1930s when the concept of food allergies became more widely accepted. One of the first elimination diet protocols was the "rice diet," which involved eating only rice and water for a period of time to help alleviate digestive issues. The rice diet was later expanded to include other foods that were thought to be easier on digestion and less likely to cause an allergic reaction or sensitivity.

In the 1950s and 1960s, elimination diets became more refined as researchers began to identify more potential allergenic foods like milk, eggs, peanuts, wheat, soy, fish, and shellfish. During this time, elimination diets were used to help people with allergies, eczema, asthma, and migraine headaches.

In the 1970s, elimination diets boomed yet again as the health food movement as a whole became more popular. People began to use elimination diets not only to identify allergenic foods but also to improve overall health and well-being. Elimination diets were seen as a way to "detox" the body and remove harmful substances from the diet.

Due to the increasing number of individuals suffering from digestive complications, elimination diets are probably more popular today than ever. The objective of an elimination diet is to remove any and all foods that may contribute to digestive distress to eliminate all symptoms and allow the digestive system to rest and restore itself. The elimination period is typically followed by a reintroduction period in which foods are slowly reintroduced while monitoring symptoms in order to identify specific problem foods.

Typically, the elimination phase of most diets lasts for around 2-4 weeks or until symptoms are cleared for at least a week (this may take longer for some individuals). During the reintroduction phase, foods are brought back into the diet one by one, with some period of time between each new food; thus, the reintroduction phase can last months and will look a little different for everyone.

There are many elimination diets that exist today and it's likely that you'll experience some amount of benefit from any one of them. However, the robustness and staying power of those benefits are drastically different from protocol to protocol. Let's look at a few of the most commonly considered elimination diets:

- **Plant-based diets like vegan/vegetarian and juice cleansing**, often mistaken as effective elimination-type diets, may provide short-term benefits because they're better than the Standard American Diet, but the presence of sugar and plant toxins will result in continued digestive discomfort and the lack of animal protein will lead to nutrient deficiencies – thus preventing the gut from structural healing.
- **Paleo** is not technically an elimination diet but is often considered one. It's closer to carnivore and typically has a greater emphasis on animal protein, but the presence of fruits and vegetables may prevent paleo from helping certain people.

- **Low FODMAP** diets allow for meat, which is great, but they also allow for vegetables containing plant toxins and grains that can further damage the structure of our digestive system.
- **Autoimmune Protocol (AIP)** is another popular elimination diet that attempts to focus on removing foods that are triggering negative reactions in the gut but allows for vegetables, sweet potatoes and fruit. Again, not complete elimination of plant compounds.

This isn't to say that these aren't good strategies for improving gut health or autoimmune symptoms for some. But because they do not cut out all of the plant compounds that can disrupt gut function, there is a chance they won't work. If a leaky gut is present, grains are going to make things worse. If the gut microbiome is in a state of dysbiosis, feeding fiber to the bad bacteria is not going to help.

This is where carnivore comes in.

The Carnivore Diet as an Elimination Diet

Of course, the carnivore diet can be considered an elimination diet because you eliminate nearly all foods. As we highlighted in the last chapter, what makes the carnivore diet superior is that it not only removes all of the foods that can trigger digestive issues but it also provides ample nutrients and, most importantly, nutrients that *repair* the gut. The same cannot be said for most other elimination diets.

This is why we created the Carnivore Reset. It's a program that is designed specifically with gut health in mind. The premise of this program is optimizing elimination to allow for digestive restoration combined with the strategic consumption of animal-based foods that strengthen the gut—a complete reset for your digestive system. Are you ready to dive in?

What to Eat

In Chapter 4, we covered what the typical carnivore diet looks like, and it's not overly complicated; you simply eat food that comes from animals.

For individuals who are using carnivore simply to lose weight, cut some bloating, reduce a little joint pain, or just improve overall wellness, this general version of carnivore is likely the perfect fit. Simply stick to the foods in the food pyramid in Chapter 4, or check out the complete carnivore food list in the Resources section at the end of this book, and you are good to go.

However, if you are dealing with more severe digestive issues or autoimmune complications, your carnivore approach may need to be adjusted a bit. That's what we did with the Carnivore Reset protocol.

What makes the Carnivore Reset protocol different from other general versions of carnivore is that it follows a stepwise approach that starts with only foods that have no chance of disrupting gut function and strengthen the gut before progressing to adding other animal-based foods like eggs and dairy to test your sensitivities to these foods in a state of better digestive strength and eventually transitioning to a reintroduction phase where you can start to incorporate non-animal-based foods looking for the foods that trigger reactions and that are likely better to be completely cut out of your diet for the long haul.

Here is a summary of what you need to know for the Carnivore Reset:

Meat Choice:

In the first week of the program, we recommend sticking with only red meat. If you recall from Chapter 3, ruminant animals have that unique digestion that allows them to produce not only more nutrient-dense meat but also filter out any compounds found in the animal's plant-based diet that could make it into our bodies and prevent a complete gut reset. Pork, poultry, and seafood don't have these same capabilities.

After the first week, you can start to incorporate pork, poultry, and fish into your diet, but just know that we still recommend limiting the consumption of these other meats and prioritizing red meat because of its superior nutrient density and gut-restorative properties.

Dairy

If you recall, there are several reasons for sensitivities to dairy. Dairy contains proteins and sugars that certain individuals can be sensitive to, especially in a state of compromised gut function. For this reason, we have cut dairy out of the beginning of the protocol.

Dairy can offer a ton of nutrients, and fermented dairy can even be beneficial to the gut, so later in the protocol, we will recommend that you try reintroducing dairy, but remember that another reason why individuals struggle with dairy consumption is due to the sources which can include ultra-processed forms that either have added ingredients that can disrupt gut function or are stripped of enzymes that assist in digestion. Thus, when it does come time to reintroduce dairy, sourcing is important.

When we do get to the part of the protocol where we reintroduce dairy, we recommend starting with fermented dairy first. Remember that part of the benefit of this protocol is starving off any potential harmful bacteria in the gut. However, it is also important to replace these with beneficial bacteria, which can be provided by fermented dairy foods like like yogurt, kefir, sauerkraut, kimchi, kombucha, an fermented cheeses.

Eggs

Eggs are also eliminated for the first couple of weeks of the reset, again not because they're unhealthy, but because it's common for individuals with digestive issues to have sensitivities to eggs.

Eggs are a true superfood, though, and the goal is to be able to consume them for their benefits without the negatives, which may be possible after gut function is restored. For this reason, eggs will be reintroduced later in the program via egg yolks first (to avoid those proteins found in egg whites). Then, we'll reintroduce the whole egg. Pay attention to how you feel when eggs are reintroduced, especially whole eggs. If you find you're experiencing flare-ups, discomfort, or any other adverse side effects, egg whites are likely causing the issue. In that case, continue avoiding them until your digestive system has more time to repair itself, and then consider trying again.

Coffee

We haven't talked about coffee yet, and coffee is no doubt another heavily debated topic in the health world, especially among carnivore dieters. Many carnivore purists will say that anything from a plant is out, so coffee is to be avoided. We'll be honest: we can handle some self-induced pain, but we're drawing the line at completely cutting out coffee forever if possible.

That said, it's crucial to address the concerns surrounding coffee, particularly regarding mold and other toxins. Coffee beans can sometimes contain mycotoxins, a form of mold, which can potentially impact gut health, contributing to issues like inflammation and digestive discomfort. These concerns are especially relevant for individuals with heightened sensitivity to molds and toxins.

If you have a known aversion to coffee, you should ditch it. Otherwise, in this program, we suggest simply eliminating it for the first 1-2 weeks of the elimination phase. If you're unsure if you're sensitive to coffee, you'll find out when you reintroduce coffee after those two weeks. Should you notice any adverse effects upon its reintroduction, it may be linked to these mold or toxin sensitivities. If you know you feel great drinking coffee, then you can consider keeping it in for the entire four weeks. The key is to be honest with yourself.

If you're drinking coffee, aim to minimize the risk of mycotoxin exposure by considering the following tips:

- **Look for Wet-Processed or Washed Coffees:** These coffee beans are processed with water immediately after harvesting, which can help in reducing mold growth.
- **Single-Origin Coffee:** Coffees sourced from a single location or farm are often more carefully monitored and can have lower mycotoxin levels compared to blends from multiple regions.
- **Roasting Level:** Darker roasts may reduce mycotoxin levels, but this is not a foolproof method.
- **Storage and Freshness:** Purchase coffee in small batches to ensure freshness. Store it in a cool, dry place to prevent mold growth.
- **Buy Whole-Bean:** Preground coffee has more exposure to air and moisture, increasing the risk of mold. Opt for whole beans and when you are ready to make coffee, do the grinding yourself. Plus, the coffee tastes better this way!
- **Transparent Suppliers:** Choose coffee suppliers who are transparent about their sourcing and processing methods. Some companies specifically test for mycotoxins and market their coffee as such.

Sunlight > Coffee

I know that the first week without coffee can be hard. It definitely was for Chris. But it's also worth it. To combat morning fatigue, we recommend getting outside and exposing yourself to sunlight as soon as you wake up and get a little light movement in to get some blood flowing. For Chris, that looks like going outside in the grass and doing a few pushups when he first wakes up.

The movement part is great, but the sunlight is key because it will stimulate your natural wake cycle. Our eyes have photoreceptors in them that, when exposed to sunlight, initiate a cascade of events that wake us up, including the production of cortisol, which suppresses melatonin from our previous night's sleep.

Getting sunlight first thing in the morning is the antidote to low morning energy and is way better than coffee....okay maybe not way better, but it's pretty damn good.

Added Ingredients
Remember, the goal of carnivore is to eliminate processed foods and the unnatural added ingredients that often come with them. During the elimination protocol, we also want to avoid as many additives as possible, which means checking food labels for hidden sugar and vegetable oils (especially important for dairy) and being mindful of processed meat intake due to ingredients like nitrates, which can be tough on the gut.

We also strongly advise limiting or cutting out added sweeteners, even non-glycemic ones, during the elimination phase. In general, natural sweeteners like monk fruit and stevia are fine, but if you have impaired digestive health, you may find that these are disruptive to your gut, so giving yourself a break from them can be helpful for rest and repair.

Spices

We talked about spices a bit in Chapter 4, and while it may seem a bit extreme, some individuals can have negative reactions to even small amounts of spices. For this reason, we recommend removing spices for at least the first couple of weeks and sticking to just salt for your meat.

Remember, this does not have to be a forever thing. Once you've given your digestive system a rest from plant compounds, you may be able to reintroduce spices and incorporate them to add more flavor to your carnivore cooking. If you do this, you're still following a carnivore diet, even if social media influencers tell you you're not.

Intermittent Fasting

Many carnivore dieters naturally progress to intermittent fasting due to the satiety experienced on this diet. Intermittent fasting offers many additional health benefits, including benefits to your digestive system. Research shows that some foods can take 14+ hours to be completely digested, meaning if you eat later at night, early in the morning, and snack throughout the day, you're keeping your digestive system working around the clock. This can cause your digestive system to burn out like you would if you had to work your job around the clock.

For this reason, we have strategically implemented fasting windows into the Reset protocol so you can experience the benefit of digestive rest and improved nutrient absorption during your feeding window. This may look a lot different from your typical intermittent fasting schedule, where you don't eat until noon every day. Instead, we will be recommending that you eat breakfast, skip lunch, eat dinner, and wait 12-14 hours after your dinner before you have your breakfast the next day.

Keep in mind that if you find this approach to be unbearable, especially at first, feel free to ditch it and opt for as many meals as required to feel satiated as long as you are sticking to the approved foods. As you progress with carnivore, if you find that you are not hungry in the morning and would like to follow a more traditional intermittent fasting approach, feel free to do what comes naturally to you.

It's important to remember that intermittent fasting does typically induce a calorie deficit, and sometimes it can easily lead to severe calorie restriction. While this is okay in the short-term, long term it's not ideal. If you incorporate fasting, be mindful of your calorie intake and make sure to adjust your calories according to your goals.

Macros & Calories

Whenever you choose a diet, you should do so with a primary goal in mind. The point of this program is to reset your gut. While weight loss and muscle gain can be pleasant "side effects" of the Carnivore Reset, they're not the primary goal of this program, which is why we aren't going to overly concern ourselves with macros or calories. Instead, we recommend focusing on eating to satiety. Many find that on carnivore, this naturally leads to a calorie deficit, and if it does, that's okay. There's some healing in that, too.

We don't recommend tracking for this program because most people find it annoying, and it can become a point of friction that may impact adherence. If you like tracking because it holds you accountable, feel free to track away and get an idea of your daily macros and calories. While you don't need to optimize them on this program, this knowledge can help you optimize your macros later in your health journey.

Carnivore Supplements

The boom in carnivore popularity has created a rush of companies trying to spin up supplements to sell to carnivore dieters, some of which are great and others of which are unnecessary or potentially counterproductive. We'll help you sift through the noise.

Since most supplements aren't exclusively animal-based, many carnivore enthusiasts will recommend against them. We have a slightly different perspective. Supplements are meant to fill in gaps in your diet. If a supplement is providing you with a useful nutrient you aren't otherwise getting or helping you reach a health goal, then we think it's worth taking, even on a carnivore diet.

That being said, due to the nutrient density of a proper carnivore diet, there aren't many supplements that are essential, but there are a few we think are worth considering (recommended supplements) and others that we think are okay if you want to take them (approved supplements).

Recommended Supplements

Electrolytes
We recommend electrolytes on any low-carb diet because low-carb diets induce a state of low blood sugar and insulin levels, which increases water excretion, resulting in dehydration and electrolyte deficiencies. Exercise and sweating also deplete electrolytes. Electrolytes play a key role in thousands of bodily processes, and side effects can range from brain fog and muscle cramps to anxiety and digestive issues. Many of which new carnivore dieters will report experiencing if not properly accounted for.

Electrolytes can be found in whole food forms, but most of the sources are not carnivore. You may be wondering how our meat-eating ancestors were able to replenish electrolytes, and the answer is that they drank blood. Since we doubt you are going to do that, we recommend supplementing with electrolyte products that contain sodium, magnesium, and potassium, which can be found in capsule or powder form. Typically, powder contains more efficacious doses, but most powders are flavored, so they aren't fully carnivore. However, the amount of other ingredients in these powders is often very small and unlikely to cause a problem in most people. Ultimately, the benefits of electrolytes outweigh the downsides of the powders, so if you aren't sensitive to the ingredients in these products, it might be worth it to give them a try.

Collagen

Collagen is the most abundant protein in the human body and is found throughout our skin, bones, and connective tissues. Our bodies actually produce collagen naturally, but as we age, our natural production slows down, which can increase the demand for supplemental collagen.

While collagen is often touted for its benefits on hair, skin, and nail health, it also plays a big role in gut health. Specifically, the amino acids found in collagen support the structure and function of the gut lining, which means that supplementing with this protein can help with gut repair.

Most collagen supplements are not 100% carnivore, so we recommend avoiding this supplement for the first two weeks of the program. From there, incorporating a clean version can help enhance your gut recovery period.

Bone Broth

Bone broth has long been touted for its many benefits, especially for gut health. Made by simmering animal bones, this nutrient-rich liquid is a great source of amino acids, collagen, and gelatin. These components work together to support the health of the gut by nourishing the intestinal lining and supporting the growth of beneficial gut bacteria.

The amino acids and collagen in bone broth help to repair damage to the intestinal wall, which combats leaky gut. The gelatin found in bone broth is a form of collagen that helps to form a protective layer over the gut lining, improving digestion and reducing inflammation. It also supports the growth of healthy gut bacteria.

Homemade Bone Broth

Bone broth has become so popular that you can now find it on the shelves at many grocery stores. The only problem with this bone broth is that it can be a bit pricy. Since you are going to be eating a lot of meat, if you find yourself eating a lot of bone-in cuts, save your bones and follow this recipe to make your own bone broth at home. You'll find that it tastes way better, too!

Ingredients:
- 2-3 pounds of mixed bones
- 2 tablespoons apple cider vinegar (helps extract nutrients from the bones)
- Water (enough to cover the bones)

Instructions:
- **Prepare the Bones**: If using beef bones, you may opt to roast them first for a deeper flavor. Preheat your oven to 400°F (200°C), place the bones on a baking sheet, and roast for 30 minutes. For chicken or turkey bones, roasting is optional.
- **Place Bones in a Large Pot**: Transfer the bones to a large stockpot. Add apple cider vinegar and enough water to completely cover the bones by an inch or two.
- **Slowly Bring to a Boil**: Heat the pot over medium-high heat and gradually bring to a gentle boil. Reduce any heat as necessary to maintain a low simmer.
- **Simmer the Broth**: Allow the broth to simmer gently. The cooking time should ideally be between 12-24 hours for beef bones and 6-12 hours for chicken or turkey bones. The longer you simmer, the richer and more flavorful the broth will be.
- **Skim the Broth**: Periodically skim off any foam or impurities that rise to the surface with a spoon or ladle.
- **Strain and Cool**: After the simmering process, remove the pot from heat. Strain the broth using a fine-mesh strainer or cheesecloth to remove all the bone pieces and any solid residue.
- **Store the Broth**: Allow the broth to cool to room temperature. Once cooled, you can refrigerate it for up to 5 days or freeze it in smaller batches for long-term use.
- Optional: During carnivore, you will probably want to keep this recipe to just bones, but after carnivore, feel free to add seasoning, herbs, and other vegetables to add more flavor.

Vitamin D3

Vitamin D has increased in popularity over the last few years due to its role in immune health, but this vitamin is important for many aspects of health, ranging from hormone levels to bone health and even gut health.

Remember, vitamin D can come in the form of D2 or D3, but D3 is more effective at raising blood levels of vitamin D. Vitamin D3 can help reduce inflammation in the gut and improve the integrity of the gut lining. Additionally, vitamin D3 can promote the growth of beneficial gut bacteria.

While it's possible to get vitamin D3 from sun exposure and certain foods, research estimates that somewhere between 40% and 70% of the population is deficient in vitamin D, which is why it would be beneficial to add this supplement to your routine, especially if you live in an area or a time of the year where access to sunlight is limited.

Vitamin D is a fat-soluble vitamin, which means that it requires fat for absorption, which is why vitamin D supplements incorporate a fat source. The problem is that many companies use seed oils, so be sure to check the ingredient label to avoid this.

The current guidelines for vitamin D intake recommend a daily dosage of 400–800 IU. However, this range is likely too low for most adults, especially those living in areas of reduced sun exposure. A daily dose of 1,000–2,000 IU of vitamin D3 is generally adequate to fulfill the requirements of the majority of individuals, but in cases where more severe deficiencies exist, a dosage guideline could be between 20–80 IU per kilogram of body weight.

The Upper Tolerable Intake Level is established at 4,000 IU daily in the United States and Canada. It's thought that this could actually be much higher at 10,000 IU per day, but comprehensive data regarding the health impacts of dosages around this higher level is somewhat limited.

K2
Vitamin K is less well-known than some of its counterparts, but it plays a vital role in many aspects of our health, including gut health. Vitamin K supports gut health by promoting the growth of beneficial gut bacteria and regulating inflammation in the gut. Vitamin K can also support the production of essential proteins necessary for maintaining the integrity of the gut lining.

Vitamin K exists in multiple forms, referred to as vitamers. These forms include phylloquinones (vitamin K1) and menaquinones (vitamin K2), with vitamin K2 further subdivided into various vitamers, denoted as MK-x.

Vitamin K2 is found in fermented foods and meat and is considered superior to K1, primarily found in plants, because of better absorption and distribution throughout the body and its ability to work synergistically with D3.

In the case of short-chain menaquinones, specifically MK-4, the minimal effective dosage starts at 1,500mcg. Higher dosages, up to 45mg (45,000mcg), have been used safely in intensive dosing regimens. For longer-chain menaquinones, such as MK-7, MK-8, and MK-9, the effective dose ranges from 90 to 360mcg. More research is necessary to establish the optimal upper dosage for MK-7.

Vitamin K2 is also a fat-soluble vitamin, so similar to D3, be sure to take it with dietary fat and be sure to check the label to avoid seed oils.

Approved Supplements

Organ meat capsules
Organ meat capsules have become very popular due to the unpleasant taste of organs in whole-food form. Organ meat capsules are made with desiccated beef organs. Desiccated means to dry out, so to make these supplements, organs are freeze-dried and ground into a fine powder and then encapsulated in a gelatin or vegetable-based capsule. If you choose to take organ supplements, gelatin-based would be the most carnivore.

The idea behind this freeze-drying process is that it preserves the key nutrients found in organ meat. We have always been a bit skeptical of how much is preserved, but many companies selling these supplements are using manufacturers that have quality control measures in place to ensure purity and potency. For this reason, this supplement might be a great addition to your carnivore diet, especially if you refuse to eat organ meat in its whole-food form. Again, we think you should get used to tasting bad things, but if you're thinking, "Hey, F you, buddy," then go ahead and get the capsules.

Protein Powder
If you are struggling to get enough protein in your carnivore diet or have increased protein demands from exercise, protein powder can be a good addition to your carnivore diet. Protein powders do typically contain some non-carnivore ingredients, and some brands contain a ton of junk, so reading the labels is essential.

The protein in protein powders can come from beef, whey, egg, or various plants. Obviously, plant-based protein is out. Egg and whey (which comes from dairy) should be avoided during the elimination phase of this program to prevent any sensitivities to the proteins and sugars that come from these sources. Beef protein is your best option for The Carnivore Reset.

Fish Oil

Fish oil may be helpful on a carnivore diet to further drive up omega-3 fatty acid intake, which is beneficial for keeping inflammation in check. You can get plenty of omega-3 fatty acids in your diet through grass-fed red meat and fatty fish, but if you feel you aren't getting enough, feel free to reach for a supplement. Remember that animal sources of omega-3 are far superior to plant-based sources, and be sure to check the label to avoid getting a product that uses seed oils.

Creatine

Creatine is an amino acid found in meat that's essential to many functions in the human body. The research on creatine for gut health isn't incredibly robust, but there is some evidence that it could support beneficial bacteria and strengthen the integrity of the gut lining. Regardless, this amino acid is one of the most research-backed supplements and can provide a range of benefits, from increasing strength and muscle mass to improving acute and long-term cognitive function.

Red meat is rich in creatine, but there are enough benefits from this amino acid that we see no reason not to include this as a supplement as well. 5-10g of creatine monohydrate will do the trick. It's cheap and tasteless! Check out Cynthia and Chris's favorite creatine at https://cynthiathurlow.com/new-shop/creatine-order/.

Disclaimer: The following information is a recommendation for using a carnivore diet as an elimination diet. Note that these recommendations are not meant to treat any medical condition or be interpreted as a prescription. If you choose to follow carnivore as an elimination diet, use the following information to simply help guide you along the way!

The Carnivore Reset Protocol

Remember, the Carnivore Reset protocol was created specifically for digestive health. It's not just general carnivore. This protocol consists of a strategic starting point and progression that will give your digestive system the opportunity to rest while also providing it with the nutrients it needs for repair.

In other words, this protocol is made specifically for those dealing with more severe gut and autoimmune complications requiring a more strict/ intense program. For those who are dealing with less severe health complications, a general carnivore diet may be all that is required. This approach is still a great way to "reset" your health and help with weight loss, reduce inflammation, improve gut health, boost mood, and increase energy. To follow this form of carnivore, which we will refer to as the **Carnivore Reset Lite**, check out the Resources section at the end of the book, where you will find a general carnivore diet list. To follow this version of carnivore, simply stick to the foods on this list, and you will be on your way to health improvements.

If you have decided that the full Carnivore Reset program is for you, let's jump into it. The protocol is broken down into three phases:
1. Reset
2. Animal-Based Reintroduction
3. Plant-Based Reintroduction

Here is a brief breakdown of each phase of the protocol.

Phase 1: Reset

This phase of the protocol focuses primarily on the two major components of digestive reset that we have discussed throughout this book:

• Digestive Rest
• Gut Restoration

In this phase, you will remove all foods that could possibly trigger digestive or inflammatory responses, which means you'll be eating just meat. This phase will last two weeks and will start with a week of just eating ruminant meat, followed by a week of incorporating other meat sources like pork, poultry, and seafood.

During this phase of the protocol, we also recommend assisting your digestive reset by:
- Eating only two meals per day (breakfast and dinner)
- Wait at least 12 hours between dinner and breakfast the next day
- Daily consumption of bone broth

Reintroduction Phases

The reintroduction part of this protocol is broken into two phases because you will be introducing foods that are animal-based, like dairy and eggs, and then you will be reintroducing plant-based foods to determine where your greatest sensitivities are.

The reintroduction phase of any elimination diet can be challenging, so let's breakdown the proper way to reintroduce foods to make it a little easier for you.

Reintroduction Approach

To really get to the bottom of your source of digestive distress, you have to take a scientific approach when you reintroduce foods so you can better evaluate the impact certain foods are having on your health. If you add back multiple foods at once or don't give yourself enough time between introducing new foods, it will be harder to decipher which foods are causing a reaction in your body. This part of the protocol is important because it will help set the framework for how you can eat without dealing with digestive complications moving forward.

Here's how this approach should look:

- Choose one food at a time that you want to reintroduce into your current carnivore diet and consume it every day (1-2x per day), in amounts you would typically consume, and do so for at least three consecutive days. It's important that you only introduce the food itself, not in a dish with several other ingredients.
- Keep a journal and write down how you feel after consuming this food. Be as detailed as you can - how's your digestion? Are you bloated? Do you have a headache? Do you feel lethargic? How's your skin? Do you feel energized? Keep note of everything!
- If a food seems to agree with you, keep it in your diet if you wish.

- If it does not agree with you and you are experiencing digestive symptoms, headaches, skin issues, etc., cut it out and return to the carnivore diet food list for at least 3-days before testing a new food.
- Repeat the steps above until you've tested all the foods you want to.
- This phase can be as long as you make it, depending on how many foods you choose to test. You might have a hunch about certain foods being problematic that you now have the opportunity to test your tolerance for or others you are confident you don't have problems with that you will add back in once you're done testing everything.

REINTRODUCTION SCHEDULE

	SUN	MON	TUE	WED	THU	FRI	SAT
1 WEEK	Add 1 Food	Monitor Your Symptoms	Add 1 Food	Monitor Your Symptoms		Add 1 Food	
2 WEEK	Monitor Your Symptoms	Add 1 Food	Monitor Your Symptoms		Add 1 Food	Monitor Your Symptoms	
3 WEEK	Monitor Your Symptoms	Add 1 Food	Monitor Your Symptoms		Add 1 Food	Monitor Your Symptoms	

Reintroduction Example - Milk

Here is a brief example of how you would reintroduce and assess dairy.
- Continue eating the foods you have been eating with the addition of milk.
- For three days in a row, consume a normal serving of milk twice per day, each day. Record how you feel after each serving and throughout the three days.
- If you have no reactions, milk can be a part of your new baseline diet for introducing other foods.
- If you have reactions, cut it out and return to an all-meat diet for the next 3-days to reset before trying a new food.
- Continue on like this, testing new foods every 3-6 days.

Phase 2: Animal-Based Reintroduction

This phase of the protocol focuses on reintroducing nutrient rich animal based foods that still contain compounds that you may be sensitive too. During this phase of the protocol, you are still 100% carnivore because you are eating only animal based foods.

This phase of the program will last four weeks where you will be introducing the following foods, one week at a time:
- Egg Yolks
- Whole Eggs
- Fermented Dairy
- General Dairy

To continue assisting with your digestive rest and recovery, we recommend sticking with the meal frequency, meal timing, and bone broth strategies from Phase 1.

Phase 3: Plant-Based Reintroduction

During this phase of the protocol, you will begin reintroducing plant-based foods, thus transitioning out of a purely carnivore diet. If you made it through the first 6 weeks of the Carnivore Reset protocol and are loving what carnivore is doing for you, feel free to push back starting this phase and continue following carnivore until it no longer serves you. However, if you came to this program because you wanted to get to the root of what's bothering you, we recommend you partake in the reintroduction phase at some point. This phase is not just about expanding your dietary repertoire; it's a critical period for gaining a deeper understanding of your body's unique responses to different foods giving you a roadmap of what a symptom free diet should look like for you moving forward.

It's important to point out that not everyone will be able to transition off of a carnivore diet. For those of you dealing with more severe autoimmune conditions, like Mikhaila was, you may find that sticking to carnivore is the only approach that keeping symptoms in remission. This phase of the protocol will help you figure out if that's the case for you or not.

How to choose which foods to introduce:

Generally, we don't recommend starting with gluten-containing foods, most grains, refined carbohydrates of any kind (flour, sugars), corn, soy, or vegetable oils for anyone, let alone someone who is dealing with moresevere gut and autoimmune issues. So, while you can certainly test these during the reintroduction phase, we recommend cutting them out of your diet entirely. If you're interested in seeing how these foods affect you personally, this reintroduction phase is really up to you, so try them if you wish.

We recommend first starting with whole foods that are known to cause trouble in some individuals, such as foods high in FODMAPs (e.g., garlic, onions, asparagus, Brussels sprouts, etc.). Remember, FODMAPS are fermentable carbohydrates that can cause unwanted digestive symptoms such as gas, bloating, and stomach pain. Beyond vegetables, experiment with different carbohydrate sources such as squashes, root vegetables, and nuts and seeds. You can even test different sweeteners like stevia, erythritol, and xylitol, and if you desire to consume grains like rice, quinoa, or oats, test these, too!

This length of this phase of the protocol is dependent on how many foods you are trying to test so really it's up to you. Remember, as you go through this phase of the protocol, keep notes on your reactions to the foods you are reintroducing. This will help you find trends that can better determine where your trouble areas are. For example, if you find that you have a terrible reaction to spinach, than it may be oxalates that are the issue for you. To test this hypothesis, reintroduce another food high in oxalates and see if you see the same type of reaction. If you do, make note that oxalate foods are not for you.

Special Note on Apple Cider Vinegar:

Apple cider vinegar (ACV) is a fermented liquid made from crushed apples that is often touted for its health benefits. It contains acetic acid, the primary component found in vinegar that gives it its sour taste and strong smell. Acetic acid is believed to aid digestion by increasing stomach acid, which can improve the breakdown and absorption of nutrients, and by its prebiotic content that may support a healthy gut microbiome.

ACV may help assist with the digestion of plant-based foods when they are added back into your diet. For this reason, we recommend first trying to add it back in with an animal-based meal to make sure the ACV itself isn't triggering a flareup. If you find your body is tolerating ACV well, try adding it in before one meal per day during the plant-based reintroduction and moving forward. **Be sure not to include ACV in a meal containing a plant-based food you are reintroducing for the first time. However, if you that food causes a reaction, give it a try again with ACV to see if the digestive assistance makes any difference.**

Carnivore Reset Protocol Overview

Weeks	Protocol
Week 1	Ruminants, Salt, Water
Week 2	Add Other Meat
Week 3	Add Egg Yolks
Week 4	Add Whole Eggs
Week 5	Add Fermented Dairy
Week 6	Add General Dairy
Week 7	Non-Carnivore Reintroduction

Important Note: It's important to be flexible within this program. If after week one you are still experiencing intense digestive or autoimmune symptoms, try sticking with week one of the protocol until you start to see some symptom resolution. As you progress through the weeks and add other foods back, be sure to pay attention to how they make you feel. If a certain food, like whole eggs or dairy, triggers any symptoms, remove it for a couple of days and try it again. After doing this a few times, if you find that a food is still triggering a negative reaction, you may need to remove this food completely, or at least for the foreseeable future.

Week 1: Reset

Food: Ruminant Animals, Salt

Drinks: Water, Bone Broth
Meal #: 2
Snacks: None/Limit
Fasting Schedule: At Least 12 hours after dinner, before breakfast

Example Day:

7 am: Breakfast: Steak
12 pm: Lunch: Bone Broth
7 pm: Dinner: Ground Beef

Week 2: Reset

Reintroduce: Pork, Poultry, Seafood
Other Food: Ruminant Animals, Salt
Drinks: Water, Bone Broth
Meal #: 2
Snacks: None/Limit
Fasting Schedule: At Least 12 hours after dinner, before breakfast

Example Day:

7 am: Breakfast: Steak
12 pm: Lunch: Bone Broth
7 pm: Dinner: Pork Loin

Week 3: Animal-Based Reintroduction

Reintroduce: Egg Yolks
Other Food: Ruminant Animals, Salt
Drinks: Water, Bone Broth, Coffee*
Meal #: 2
Snacks: None/Limit
Fasting Schedule: At Least 12 hours after dinner, before breakfast

Example Day:

7 am: Breakfast: 2-3 Egg Yolks, Ground Sausage
12 pm: Lunch: Bone Broth
7 pm: Dinner: Salmon

*Feel free to give coffee a try this week but make sure not to consume it with or too closely to eggs so you don't confuse a potential trigger.

Week 4: Animal-Based Reintroduction

Reintroduce: Whole Eggs
Other Food: Egg Yolks, Ruminant Animals, Salt
Drinks: Water, Bone Broth, Coffee
Meal #: 2
Snacks: None/Limit
Fasting Schedule: At Least 12 hours after dinner, before breakfast

Example Day:

7 am: Breakfast: 2-3 Whole Eggs, Ground Sausage
12 pm: Lunch: Bone Broth
7 pm: Dinner: Steak

Week 5: Animal-Based Reintroduction

Reintroduce: Fermented Dairy
Other Food: Whole Eggs, Ruminant Animals, Salt
Drinks: Water, Bone Broth, Coffee
Meal #: 2
Snacks: Limit
Fasting Schedule: At Least 12 hours after dinner, before breakfast

Example Day:

7 am: Breakfast: Fermented Yogurt/Kefir, Ground Sausage
12 pm: Lunch: Bone Broth
7 pm: Dinner: Ground Beef, Whole Eggs

Week 6: Animal-Based Reintroduction

Reintroduce: General Dairy
Other Food: Fermented Dairy, Whole Eggs, Ruminant Animals, Salt
Drinks: Water, Bone Broth, Coffee
Meal #: 2
Snacks: As desired

Fasting Schedule: At Least 12 hours after dinner, before breakfast

Example Day:

7 am: Breakfast: Unflavored Greek Yogurt, Uncured Bacon
12 pm: Lunch: Bone Broth
7 pm: Dinner: Steak, Whole Eggs

Week 7+: Plant-Based Reintroduction

Reintroduce: ??
Other Food: Dairy, Whole Eggs, Ruminant Animals, Salt
Drinks: Water, Bone Broth, Coffee, ACV
Meal #: 2
Snacks: As desired
Fasting Schedule: At Least 12 hours after dinner, before breakfast

Example Day:

7 am: Breakfast: ACV, Eggs, Greek Yogurt
12 pm: Lunch: Bone Broth
7 pm: Dinner: Burger Patty, Cheese, Uncured Bacon, Side of Asparagus

Nutrition Moving Forward

Unless you have more severe autoimmune symptoms persisting when you reintroduce plant based foods, it's unlikely that you are going to follow a carnivore diet for life, but that doesn't mean you should return to the diet that caused you all the issues in the first place. So, what should you eat? After all of this is completed, you should have a better idea of the foods that make you feel great and those that make you feel worse. That's a great place to start.

The list of foods that you know you have no reactions to should comprise the bulk of your diet, and you should make an effort to avoid those that cause discomfort or any other unwanted side effects.

Now that you have experience with a carnivore diet and feel comfortable with it, you may choose to use it as a tool, incorporating the lessons you learned whenever your body feels it needs a reset, whether that be a single meal, a day, a week, or a month.

We strongly recommend avoiding processed foods after you complete this protocol and instead encourage a focus on whole foods. We are also advocates of low-carbohydrate diets for long-term health. Check out the General Food List For Life in the Resource section to see more about what eating like this looks like. Remember, part of why carnivore works is because of what it is not. Use this understanding to shape your nutrition for the rest of you life.

Wrap Up/Coaching

If you made it through this book and haven't started the protocol yet, the time is now. You've dealt with digestive issues for far too long to wait any longer.

Use this book as a resource and leverage the information to take action on restoring your digestive health. If you find that you're a bit intimidated and would like additional support, visit carnivorereset.com, and enroll in our coaching program, where we will walk you step-by-step through carnivore and tailor the diet specifically to your needs!

Resources

Full Carnivore Food List

Meats
* Beef: Steaks, roasts, ribs, ground beef
* Pork: Chops, bacon, ham, pork belly
* Lamb: Chops, leg of lamb, ground lamb
* Chicken: Breast, thighs, wings, drumsticks
* Turkey: Whole turkey, ground turkey, turkey breast
* Game Meats: Venison, bison, elk, rabbit

Organ Meats
* Liver: Beef, chicken, or lamb liver
* Heart: Beef, chicken, or lamb heart
* Kidney: Beef, pork, or lamb kidney
* Tongue: Beef or lamb tongue
* Brain: Typically from lamb or pork
* Sweetbreads: Thymus or pancreas, usually from lamb or veal

Seafood
- Fish: Salmon, trout, mackerel, sardines, tuna, herring
- Shellfish: Shrimp, crab, lobster, oysters, mussels, clams
- Other Seafoods: Octopus, squid, scallops

Eggs and Dairy (Optional)
- Eggs: Chicken, duck, quail
- Dairy: Butter, ghee, heavy cream (for those who tolerate dairy well)
- Cheese: Hard and soft cheeses (preferably full-fat and minimally processed)

Fats and Oils (Animal-Based)
- Tallow: Rendered beef fat
- Lard: Rendered pork fat
- Duck Fat: Rendered duck fat
- Butter and Ghee: Preferably from grass-fed sources

Bone Products
- Bone Broth: Made from beef, chicken, or fish bones
- Bone Marrow: Often consumed directly from roasted bones

General Food List For Life

Everything included in the carnivore food list

+

Fruits and Vegetables
- Green leafy vegetables: kale, spinach, collard greens, bok choy, arugula, lettuce, etc.
- Cruciferous vegetables: broccoli, cauliflower, Brussels sprouts, cabbage, etc.
- Asparagus
- Mushrooms
- Onions, green onions, shallots, leeks etc.
- Avocado
- Zucchini
- Bell peppers

- Eggplant
- Tomatoes
- Spaghetti squash
- Fermented Foods (e.g., sauerkraut, kimchee, pickles)

Oils and Fats
- Grass-fed butter and ghee
- Tallow
- Lard
- Virgin coconut oil (unrefined)
- Extra-virgin olive oil
- Avocado oil

Herbs and Spices
- Garlic (fresh or powdered)
- Rosemary
- Oregano
- Bay leaves
- Cinnamon
- Thyme
- Cloves
- Cumin

In moderation
- Nuts and seeds
- Low-sugar berries - wild blueberries, strawberries, blackberries, raspberries
- Nuts - watch out for these, but some are ok
- Peanuts (are actually legumes)

Condiments
- Mustard
- Hot sauce (sugar-free)
- Coconut Aminos
- Wheat-free tamari
- Sea salt
- Vinegar
- Avocado or olive oil-based dressings (sugar-free)

Foods to Avoid
- Sugars - white sugar, brown sugar, honey, agave, coconut sugar,

high fructose corn syrup, etc.
* Refined grains - wheat flour, rice flour, corn meal, oat flour, etc.
* Vegetable oils - canola oil, soybean oil, sunflower oil, safflower oil, corn oil, peanut oil, grapeseed oil, etc.
* Packaged foods - crackers, cereal, breads, chips, etc.
* Sauces and condiments with sugar - ketchup, marinades, salad dressings, etc.
* Sugar-sweetened beverages

FAQ/Common Issues

Why Am I Experiencing Diarrhea/Loose Stools On Carnivore?

Experiencing diarrhea or loose stools on a carnivore diet can be due to the body adjusting to higher fat intake, changes in gut microbiota, and the transition to a lower fiber diet. Initially, your digestive system may struggle to produce enough bile and enzymes to digest the increased fat, leading to looser stools. In most cases, symptoms resolve themselves but to help alleviate, focus on staying well-hydrated. If symptoms persist, consulting with a healthcare professional is recommended to ensure the diet is suitable for your individual health needs.

Is The Carnivore Diet Nutritionally Complete?

The carnivore diet can provide the most essential nutrients, especially if a variety of meats, including organ meats, are consumed. Organ meats are particularly nutrient-dense. However, the diet may be low in certain nutrients found primarily in plants, such as fiber and vitamin C.

Can I Follow The Carnivore Diet Long-Term?

The long-term sustainability of the carnivore diet is a subject of debate among nutrition experts. There's no definitive evidence that suggests that long-term carnivore dieting is dangerous, and many individuals have found success following this diet long-term. However, if the body is able to tolerate eating plants, returning to an omnivorous diet is the way to go.

Is The Carnivore Diet Safe For People With High Cholesterol?

The impact of the carnivore diet on cholesterol levels can vary. Some people experience an increase in cholesterol levels, while others do not. Outside of the context of this book, it's worth noting that our current understanding of cholesterol levels is based on decades of misunderstanding this important nutrient and its role in health and disease. More research is emerging, demonstrating that cholesterol itself is a weak predictor of cardiovascular disease, and in fact, when cholesterol levels are too low, it can be dangerous. Additionally, carnivore leads to other improvements in metabolic health like decreased inflammation and insulin resistance, which are more significant predictors of CVD risk than cholesterol, and reduce the capacity for cholesterol to become problematic.

Regardless, it's essential to have your cholesterol levels monitored and to discuss any changes with a healthcare provider, especially if you have a history of heart disease.

How Do I Get Enough Vitamins And Minerals?

Meat is loaded with vitamins and minerals, especially organ meat, fatty fish, and grass-fed beef. Eating a variety of these foods is the key to getting enough vitamins and minerals in your diet. If certain vitamin deficiencies present themselves, supplementation is also a great option.

How Do I Navigate Social Settings And Dining Out?

Social gatherings and dining out can be challenging on a strict carnivore diet. When dining out, opt for simple meat-based dishes like steaks or grilled fish. For social events, consider eating beforehand or being okay with just opting for the available protein.

Can I Do Intense Exercise On A Carnivore Diet?

Yes, you can engage in intense exercise while on a carnivore diet, and we encourage you to do so! Ensure you're consuming enough calories to fuel your activity, especially focusing on protein for muscle repair and recovery. Listen to your body and adjust your food intake based on your energy needs. Consider supplementing with electrolytes to support hydration and mineral levels depleted during exercise.

Is It Normal To Feel Fatigue And Weakness?

Some individuals may experience fatigue or weakness when they first start the carnivore diet, often referred to as "keto flu." This is usually temporary as your body adapts to using fat for energy. Most often, signs of keto flu are related to dehydration and electrolyte deficiencies, so staying hydrated, ensuring adequate salt intake, and supplementing with electrolytes can help mitigate these symptoms.

Why Am I Experiencing Bad Breath And Body Odor Changes?

Some people on the carnivore diet report experiencing bad breath or a change in body odor. This can be due to the production of ketones, which are by-products of fat metabolism, or a result of toxins being released from stored fat in the fat-burning process. Maintaining good oral hygiene and staying well-hydrated can help mitigate bad breath.

What Do I Do If I Have Difficulty Meeting Caloric Needs?

Given the high satiety factor of meat, some individuals might find it challenging to consume enough calories, especially if they're active. If this is the case, consider including calorie-dense foods like fatty cuts of meat and incorporating protein shakes to increase calorie intake.

Is It Normal To Experience Increased Thirst And Urination?

Yes, it's common to experience increased thirst and urination when starting a carnivore diet, especially one that puts your body into a state of ketosis. This is due to the diuretic effect of a low-carb diet. It's important to stay hydrated and ensure adequate electrolyte intake.

How Do I Manage Cravings For Sugars and Carbs?

Cravings for sugars and carbs can occur, especially in the initial stages of the diet, as the body transitions from using glucose to fat for energy. Over time, these cravings typically diminish, so if you are experiencing them, be patient. Staying consistent with the diet, ensuring you eat enough, and staying hydrated can help manage these cravings.

Recipes

One of the charms of the carnivore diet is its simplicity – focusing on meat and animal products makes meal preparation straightforward and time-efficient. Yet, this simplicity, while appealing to many, can sometimes verge on the mundane. To infuse a bit of culinary excitement into your carnivore routine, here are a few of our favorite recipes to try.

You'll notice that many of these recipes contain spices and seasoning. While these additions can elevate the flavor profile, they may not be suitable for the initial, more restrictive phases of the Carnivore Reset program. If you're in the early stages or sensitive to certain spices, feel free to simplify these recipes by sticking to salt.

Additionally, some recipes in this section incorporate eggs and dairy. Be sure only to include eggs and dairy once you've reached the phase of the program where these foods are reintroduced.

Breakfast

Bacon or Sausage Egg Cups

Serves 4
Prep time: 5 minutes/Cook time: 18 minutes

3 tablespoons butter
10 eggs
2 teaspoons salt
1 teaspoon pepper
8 strips bacon, cooked and crumbled, or 8 oz. of sausage
½ cup shredded cheddar cheese

1. Preheat the oven to 325F. Using the butter, grease a 12-cup muffin tin thoroughly.
2. In a large bowl, whisk the eggs until scrambled. Add in the salt, pepper, bacon, and cheese. Whisk until combined. Pour the mixture into each muffin tin, distributing it evenly between the 12 cups.
3. Put the muffin tin in the oven for about 18 minutes or until browned and set. Remove and let cook a few minutes before removing. You may need to run a knife around the edges to help get them out.
4. Serve or store in an airtight container in the refrigerator for up to 3 days.

Sausage and Goat Cheese Frittata

Serves 6
Prep time: 5 minutes/Cook time: 30 minutes

1 tablespoon butter

1 pound breakfast sausage, cooked and crumbled
10 eggs
½ cup goat cheese
1 teaspoon salt
½ teaspoon pepper

1. Preheat the oven to 350F. Grease a 9-inch pie dish and set aside.
2. In a large mixing bowl, whisk the eggs, salt and pepper together. Add the sausage and goat cheese and gently mix. Put into the greased pie dish. Place in the oven and cook for about 30 minutes or until golden brown and the center is set.
3. Remove the frittata from the oven and let cool for ten minutes. Once cooled, slice into 6 equal slices.
4. Serve or store in an airtight container in the refrigerator for up to 3 days.

Chaffle Breakfast Sandwich

Serves 2
Prep time: 5 minutes/Cook time: 8 minutes

2 eggs
1 cup shredded mozzarella
4 sausage patties, cooked

1. Preheat the waffle maker according to the manufacturer's instructions.
2. In a small mixing bowl, mix together the egg and shredded cheese. Stir until well combined.
3. Once the waffle maker is heated, pour half of the batter into the waffle maker. Cook for 3-4 minutes or until golden brown. Remove and repeat with the second half of the batter.
4. Cut each waffle in half to make a top and bottom to your sandwich. Assemble each sandwich with two sausage patties.
5. Serve or store in an airtight container in the refrigerator for up to 3 days.

Egg and Bacon Roll-Ups

Serves 1
Cook time: 5 minutes

1 tablespoon butter

2 eggs, beaten
4 strips of bacon, cooked and in strips

1. Heat a medium sauté pan over medium heat.
2. In a small bowl, whisk the eggs. Add the butter to the pan and melt. Once melted, add the eggs evenly to the pan. Let the eggs set for a minute, and then, using a rubber spatula, gently lift the cooked eggs from the edges of the pan and tilt the pan to allow the uncooked eggs to flow around the edge of the pan. Once completely cooked, it will look similar to a tortilla. Slide onto a plate and place the bacon towards one end. Roll the egg around the bacon,
3. Serve or store in an airtight container in the refrigerator for up to 3 days.

Sausage Egg in a Basket

Serves 1
Prep time: 2 minutes /Cook time: 10 minutes
Dairy Free

4 ounces ground breakfast sausage
1 egg

1. Set a small sauté pan over medium heat.
2. On a plate, form the sausage into a disk. Make a 3-inch hole in the center. Be sure the sausage is about 1 inch thick all the way around so that it will cook evenly.
3. Into the hot pan, place the sausage. Cook for about 4 minutes on each side or until browned and cooked through.
4. Increase the heat to medium-high and add the egg to the center of the sausage. Cover the pan with a lid and cook to your desired doneness. If you prefer a runny yolk, cook for about 2 minutes. If you prefer your egg cooked through, cook for 4 to 5 minutes or until it is no longer runny.
5. Serve immediately or refrigerate in an airtight container for up to 3 days.

Lunch/Dinner

Bacon Scallop Skewers

Serves 1

Prep time: 5 minutes/Cook time: 12 minutes
Egg/Dairy free

4 scallops
4 slices bacon

1. Arrange bacon slices in a single layer on a disposable foil pan—Grill over medium-high, around 350F, for 3 to 5 minutes or until bacon is halfway cooked. Remove bacon from the grill and cool slightly.
2. Wrap one piece of bacon around each scallop and thread onto skewers.
3. Grill skewers over medium heat for 6 to 8 minutes or until scallops are opaque and bacon is crispy, turning occasionally.
4. Serve or store in the refrigerator in an airtight container for up to 2 days.

Bacon Wrapped Chicken Tenders

Serves 1
Prep time 15 minutes/ Cook time 30 minutes
Egg/Dairy free

1 lb chicken tenders, approximately 10 tenders
10 strips of bacon

1. Preheat the oven to 350F and line a baking sheet with parchment paper or foil.
2. Pat the chicken tenders dry with a paper towel. Wrap each tender with one slice of bacon and place seam side down on the baking sheet.
3. Place the tenders in the oven and bake for about 30 minutes or until bacon is crispy and chicken is 165F.
4. Serve or store in an airtight container in the refrigerator for up to 3 days.

Garlic Butter Steak Bites

Serves 1
Prep time: 5 minutes /Cook time: 6 minutes
Egg-Free

1 ribeye steak, cut into ½ inch cubes
2 tablespoons butter

2 teaspoons garlic powder
1 teaspoon salt
½ teaspoon pepper

1. Heat a medium sauté pan over medium-high heat.
2. Once the pan is heated, add the butter and garlic powder and move around with a spatula until melted and mixed in. Salt and pepper the steak Cubs and then add to the pan. Sear all of the sides of the steak cubes and cook until the desired temperature—about 6 minutes for well done.
3. Serve or store in an airtight container in the refrigerator for up to 3 days.

Bacon Cheeseburger Bombs

Serves 3
Prep time: 10 minutes/ Cook time: 30 minutes
Egg-Free

1 lb ground beef
2 teaspoons garlic powder
1 teaspoon onion powder
1 teaspoon salt
½ teaspoon pepper
4 ounces cheddar cheese block, cubed into 9 pieces
9 slices of bacon

1. Preheat the oven to 375F.
2. In a medium bowl, add the beef, garlic powder, onion powder, salt, and pepper and mix until combined—portion the mixture into nine evenly sized balls.
3. Flatten each ball and place a cube of cheese in the center. Form the meat around the cheese, sealing it in. Wrap each ball with a slice of bacon and place on a foil-lined baking sheet. Place in the oven and bake for 30 minutes or until the beef is cooked through and the bacon is crispy.
4. Serve or store in an airtight container in the refrigerator for up to 3 days.

Sunny Side Up Burger

1 serving
Prep 1 min./Cook 8 min.
Dairy Free
5 oz ground beef
1 egg

1. Heat a medium sauté pan over medium-high heat.
2. Form the ground beef into a patty about 1 inch thick. Add the patty to the pan and cook for about 4 minutes. Flip the patty and continue to cook for another 4 minutes. While the burger is cooking, crack your egg carefully into the pan and make a sunny-side-up egg. Once the egg whites are firm, place the egg on top of the burger to continue to cook; once the burger has finished cooking, remove it from the pan and serve.
3. If cooking for a future meal, store it in an airtight container for up to 2 days in the refrigerator.

Creamy Garlic Pork Chops

Serves 6
Prep time 5 minutes/ Cook time 15 minutes
Egg-Free

6 center-cut boneless pork chops, ½ inch thick
2 tablespoons butter
1 cup heavy whipping cream
1 oz cream cheese, room temperature
⅓ cup chicken broth
½ cup parmesan cheese
1 tablespoon Italian seasoning
1 tablespoon garlic powder
1/2 teaspoon pepper
1 teaspoon salt

1. Heat a large skillet over medium-high heat. Add the butter. When melted, add the pork chops and season with salt and pepper. Cook each side for about 4 minutes. Remove and set aside.
2. Add the chicken broth to the pan, and using a rubber spatula, scrape up all of the little bits in the pan. Then add the remaining ingredients and stir until well combined and the cheeses have melted. Add the pork chops back to a simmer for 5 minutes.

3.   Serve or store in an airtight container in the refrigerator for up to 3 days.

Organ Meat

Sautéed Beef Livers

Serves 3
Prep time: 5 minutes/ Cook time: 6 minutes
Egg-Free

1 lb beef livers livers
2 tablespoons butter

1.   In a large sauté pan over medium-high heat, melt the butter. Once hot, add the chicken livers. Sauté for about 6 minutes while moving the livers around in the pan. Once browned and firm, remove from the heat
2.   Serve or store in an airtight container in the refrigerator for up to 2 days.

Beef Heart Skewers

Serves 2
Prep time: 10 minutes/ Cook time: 8 minutes
Egg-Free

1 beef heart, 1-inch cubes
1 tablespoon butter

1.   Place three beef cubes on each skewer.
2.   Heat a large sauté pan over medium-high heat. Add the butter. Once melted, add the beef heart skewers and cook for about 4 minutes on each side until browned and firm.
3.   Serve or store in an airtight container in the refrigerator for up to 2 days.

Beef Heart/Liver Meatballs

Serves 4
Prep time: 5 minutes/ Cook time: 25 minutes
Egg/Dairy-Free

8 ounces ground beef
4 ounces ground beef heart
4 ounces of ground liver
1 teaspoon salt

1. Preheat the oven to 350F.
2. In a medium bowl, mix the ground beef, heart, and liver until well combined—season with salt. Roll the mixture into 2 inch balls and place on a foil-lined baking sheet. Place in the oven and bake for 25 minutes or until the meatballs are firm and cooked through.
3. Serve or store in an airtight container in the refrigerator for up to 3 days.

Beef Liver Pate

Serves 4
Prep time: 5 minutes/ Cook time: 2 minutes
Egg-Free

1/2 pound beef liver, sliced thin
6 tablespoons butter
1 teaspoon salt
1/2 teaspoon pepper
2 tablespoons heavy cream

1. In a large sauté pan over high heat, melt three tablespoons of butter. Add the sliced beef heart and sear for 1 minute on each side. Remove from the pan and let cool for a few minutes.
2. Transfer the liver to a food processor or blender and purée until smooth. While purring, add the remaining butter, salt, pepper, and heavy cream. Once smooth remove and place in an airtight container and refrigerate for at least 4 hours to let it harden.
3. Store for up to 3 days in the refrigerator.

Organ Meat Blend Recipes

Earlier, we discussed how organ meat blends are an effective way to include organ meats in your diet, minimizing their distinct taste and texture. Chris's wife's experience is a perfect example. During her pregnancy, she aimed to enrich her diet with nutrient-dense foods for their son's growth and development. Initially hesitant about organ meats, they introduced her to ancestral organ meat blends from Force of Nature. They experimented with these blends in various recipes, and to their delight, she thoroughly enjoyed them. Even with an initial reluctance towards organ meats, she was able to incorporate them weekly throughout her pregnancy, thanks to the versatility and palatability of these blends.

These blends are a fantastic substitute for ground meat in numerous dishes. Beyond the carnivore diet, they can be used in tacos, stews, and more. For a strict carnivore diet, they can be great for burgers, but adding some cheese may be necessary to mask the taste further.

Here is my all-time favorite organ meat blend recipe that tastes so good even my son eats it!

Organ Meat Taco Pie

Serves 4-6
Prep time: 15 minutes/ Cook time: 30 minutes

1 lb of organ meat blend
1 cup of shredded cheddar cheese
6 large eggs
½ cup heavy cream
3 tablespoons of taco seasoning
2 cloves of minced garlic
Salt & pepper to taste

1. Preheat the oven to 350°F and grease a 9-inch glass or ceramic pie pan.
2. Cook the ground organ meat in a large skillet for about 7 minutes, breaking up clumps as much as possible
3. Stir in the taco seasoning until well combined, then transfer the beef to the prepared pie pan.
4. In a large bowl, whisk together the eggs, cream, garlic, salt, and pepper. Pour over beef in the pan.
5. Sprinkle with the shredded cheese and bake for 30 minutes or until the center is cooked (test with a knife).

Snacks

Beef Jerky

Serves 3
Prep time: 10 minutes/Cook time: 3-5 hours
Egg/Dairy Free

1 pound 97/3 ground beef
1 teaspoon onion powder
1 teaspoon pepper
1 teaspoon garlic powder
¼ teaspoon curing salt

1. Preheat the oven to 200F.
2. In a large bowl, mix all of the ingredients until well combined. Add the mixture to a large ziplock bag and cut a ¼ inch hole in the corner. On a foil-lined baking sheet or a baking sheet with a rack, pipe 4-inch strips in a row until you use all of the meat. Put the baking sheet in the oven. After 3 hours, check the jerky. When the jerky bends but doesn't break in half, it is done. Continue to cook if the jerky breaks when you bend it. Once done, remove from the oven and let cool for 2 hours before storing.
3. Store in an airtight container for a week.

Egg Salad

Serves 1
Prep time: 20 minutes/Cook time: 15 minutes

3 eggs
2 tablespoons sour cream
1 tablespoon cream cheese, softened
1 teaspoon salt
½ teaspoon pepper
1 teaspoon onion powder

1. Place eggs in a medium saucepan and cover with cold water. Place on the stove over high heat and bring to a boil. Cover with a lid and let stand for 12 minutes. Remove from hot water and place in a bowl with ice water to cool down.

2. Once cooled, peel and chop the eggs and place them in a bowl with the remaining ingredients. Mix in the remaining ingredients until combined.
3. Serve or store in an airtight container in the refrigerator for up to 3 days.

Chicken Bacon and Cheese Pinwheels

Serves 1
Prep time: 5 minutes/Cook time: 8 minutes
Egg-Free

½ cup shredded mozzarella
¼ cup diced chicken, cooked
2 slices of bacon, cooked and crumbled

1. Place a medium nonstick sauté pan over medium-high heat.
2. Once the pan is hot, spread the cheese evenly into a 5-inch circle. Once it starts to melt, sprinkle the chicken and bacon evenly on top of the cheese. Once the cheese becomes browned on the bottom, slide out of the pan onto a plate and let cool for a minute. Roll the cheese like you would roll up a map. Once rolled, slice into half-inch circles.
3. Serve or store in the refrigerator in an airtight container for up to 3 days.

Chicken Bacon and Cheese Pinwheels

Serves 1
Prep time: 5 minutes/Cook time: 8 minutes
Egg-Free

½ cup shredded mozzarella
¼ cup diced chicken, cooked
2 slices of bacon, cooked and crumbled

1. Place a medium nonstick sauté pan over medium-high heat.
2. Once the pan is hot, spread the cheese evenly into a 5-inch circle. Once it starts to melt, sprinkle the chicken and bacon evenly on top of the cheese. Once the cheese becomes brown on the bottom, slide it out of the pan onto a plate and let cool for a minute. Roll the

cheese like you would roll up a map. Once rolled, slice into half-inch circles.
3. Serve or store in the refrigerator in an airtight container for up to 3 days.

Salmon and Shrimp Roll-Ups

Serves 2
Prep time: 8 minutes
Egg-Free

3 ounces sliced smoked salmon
4 ounces shrimp, cooked, peeled, deveined, and cold
2 ounces cream cheese, softened
2 tsp dried dill

1. Place a piece of smoked salmon on a cutting board. Gently spread a thin layer of cream cheese on top of the salmon. Lightly sprinkle with a little of the dill. Place about three shrimp in a row on top of the cream cheese. Then, gently roll the salmon around the shrimp. Slice into 1-inch pieces and repeat with the remaining ingredients.
2. Serve or store in the refrigerator in an airtight container for up to 2 days.

Cream Cheese Sausage Balls

Serves 3
Prep time: 5 minutes/Cook time: 25 minutes
Egg-Free

1 pound ground sausage
6 ounces cream cheese, softened
6 ounces shredded cheddar

1. Preheat the oven to 375F.
2. In a large bowl, mix all ingredients until well combined. Scoop with a small cookie scoop and roll into balls. Place the balls on a parchment-lined baking sheet and place in the preheated oven. Bake for 30 minutes or until golden brown.
3. Serve or store in the refrigerator in an airtight container for up to 3 days.`

Citations

Introduction:

1. National Institutes of Health, U.S. Department of Health and Human Services. (2009). Opportunities and challenges in digestive diseases research: Recommendations of the National Commission on Digestive Diseases. Bethesda, MD: National Institutes of Health. NIH Publication 08–6514.
2. Almario, C. V., et al. (2018). Burden of gastrointestinal symptoms in the United States: Results of a nationally representative survey of over 71,000 Americans. American Journal of Gastroenterology, 113(11), 1701–1710.

Chapter 1:

1. Fasano, A. (2020). All disease begins in the (leaky) gut: role of zonulin-mediated gut permeability in the pathogenesis of some chronic inflammatory diseases. F1000Research, 9, F1000 Faculty Rev-69.
2. Fasano, A. (2010). Leaky gut and autoimmune diseases. Clinical Reviews in Allergy & Immunology, 42(1), 71-78.
3. Michielan, A., & D'Incà, R. (2015). Intestinal Permeability in Inflammatory Bowel Disease: Pathogenesis, Clinical Evaluation, and Therapy of Leaky Gut. Mediators of Inflammation, 2015, 628157.
4. Cardoso-Silva, D., et al. (2019). Intestinal barrier function in gluten-related disorders. Nutrients, 11, 2325.
5. Nazanin, S., et al. (2018). The role of gastrointestinal permeability in food allergy. Annals of Allergy, Asthma & Immunology, 121(2), 141-142.
6. Camilleri, M., et al. (2012). Irritable bowel syndrome: methods, mechanisms, and pathophysiology. The confluence of increased permeability, inflammation, and pain in irritable bowel syndrome. American Journal of Physiology-Gastrointestinal and Liver Physiology, 303, G775-G785.
7. Teixeira, T., et al. (2012). Potential mechanisms for the emerging link between obesity and increased intestinal permeability. Nutrition Research, 32(9), 637-647.
8. Gérard, C., & Vidal, H. (2019). Impact of Gut Microbiota on Host Glycemic Control. Frontiers in Endocrinology (Lausanne), 10, 29.
9. Rowland, I., et al. (2018). Gut microbiota functions: metabolism

of nutrients and other food components. European Journal of Nutrition, 57(1), 1-24.

10. Wu, H.J., & Wu, E. (2012). The role of gut microbiota in immune homeostasis and autoimmunity. Gut Microbes, 3(1), 4-14.

11. Appleton, J. (2018). The gut-brain axis: influence of microbiota on mood and mental health. Integrative Medicine (Encinitas), 17(4), 28-32.

12. Van de Wouw, M., et al. (2017). Microbiota-gut-brain axis: modulator of host metabolism and appetite. The Journal of Nutrition, 147(5), 727-745.

13. Kelly, J.R., et al. (2015). Breaking down the barriers: the gut microbiome, intestinal permeability, and stress-related psychiatric disorders. Frontiers in Cellular Neuroscience, 9, 392.

14. David, L.A., Maurice, C.F., Carmody, R.N., et al. (2014). Diet rapidly and reproducibly alters the human gut microbiome. Nature, 505(7484), 559-563.

15. Schnorr, S.L., et al. (2014). Gut microbiome of the Hadza hunter-gatherers. Nature Communications, 5, 3654.

16. Martinez, K.B., et al. (2017). Western diets, gut dysbiosis, and metabolic diseases: Are they linked?. Gut Microbes, 8(2), 130-142.

17. Kwa, M., Plottel, C. S., Blaser, M. J., & Adams, S. (2016). The Intestinal Microbiome and Estrogen Receptor-Positive Female Breast Cancer. Journal of the National Cancer Institute, 108(8), djw029.

18. Clarke, S. F., et al. (2014). Exercise and associated dietary extremes impact on gut microbial diversity. Gut, 63(12), 1913–1920.

19. Benedict, C., Vogel, H., Jonas, W., Woting, A., Blaut, M., Schürmann, A., & Cedernaes, J. (2016). Gut microbiota and glucometabolic alterations in response to recurrent partial sleep deprivation in normal-weight young individuals. Molecular metabolism, 5(12), 1175–1186.

20. Knowles, S. R., Nelson, E. A., & Palombo, E. A. (2008). Investigating the role of perceived stress on bacterial flora activity and salivary cortisol secretion: a possible mechanism underlying susceptibility to illness. Biological psychology, 77(2), 132–137.

21. Deol, P., Ruegger, P., Logan, G. D., Shawki, A., Li, J., Mitchell, J. D., Yu, J., Piamthai, V., Radi, S. H., Hasnain, S., Borkowski, K., Newman, J. W., McCole, D. F., Nair, M. G., Hsiao, A., Borneman, J., & Sladek, F. M. (2023). Diet high in linoleic acid dysregulates the intestinal endocannabinoid system and increases susceptibility to colitis in Mice. Gut microbes, 15(1), 2229945.

22. Do, M. H., Lee, E., Oh, M. J., Kim, Y., & Park, H. Y. (2018). High-Glucose or -Fructose Diet Cause Changes of the Gut Microbiota and Metabolic Disorders in Mice without Body Weight Change. Nutrients, 10(6), 761.

23. Fajstova A, Galanova N, Coufal S, Malkova J, Kostovcik M, Cermakova M, Pelantova H, Kuzma M, Sediva B, Hudcovic T, et al. Diet Rich in Simple Sugars Promotes Pro-Inflammatory Response via Gut Microbiota Alteration and TLR4 Signaling. Cells. 2020; 9(12):2701.

24. Mutlu, E. A., Gillevet, P. M., Rangwala, H., Sikaroodi, M., Naqvi, A., Engen, P. A., Kwasny, M., Lau, C. K., & Keshavarzian, A. (2012). Colonic microbiome is altered in alcoholism. American journal of physiology. Gastrointestinal and liver physiology, 302(9), G966–G978.

25. Queipo-Ortuño, M. I., Boto-Ordóñez, M., Murri, M., Gomez-Zumaquero, J. M., Clemente-Postigo, M., Estruch, R., Cardona Diaz, F., Andrés-Lacueva, C., & Tinahones, F. J. (2012). Influence of red wine polyphenols and ethanol on the gut microbiota ecology and biochemical biomarkers. The American journal of clinical nutrition, 95(6), 1323–1334.

26. Bishehsari, F., Magno, E., Swanson, G., Desai, V., Voigt, R. M., Forsyth, C. B., & Keshavarzian, A. (2017). Alcohol and Gut-Derived Inflammation. Alcohol research : current reviews, 38(2), 163–171.

27. Elvers KT, Wilson VJ, Hammond A, et alAntibiotic-induced changes in the human gut microbiota for the most commonly prescribed antibiotics in primary care in the UK: a systematic reviewBMJ Open 2020;10:e035677. doi: 10.1136/bmjopen-2019-035677

28. Jernberg, C., Löfmark, S., Edlund, C., & Jansson, J. K. (2007). Long-term ecological impacts of antibiotic administration on the human intestinal microbiota. The ISME journal, 1(1), 56–66.

29. Ventola C. L. (2015). The antibiotic resistance crisis: part 1: causes and threats. P & T : a peer-reviewed journal for formulary management, 40(4), 277–283.

30. Cicchinelli, S., Rosa, F., Manca, F., Zanza, C., Ojetti, V., Covino, M., Candelli, M., Gasbarrini, A., Franceschi, F., & Piccioni, A. (2023). The Impact of Smoking on Microbiota: A Narrative Review. Biomedicines, 11(4), 1144.

31. Berkowitz, L., Schultz, B. M., Salazar, G. A., Pardo-Roa, C., Sebastián, V. P., Álvarez-Lobos, M. M., & Bueno, S. M. (2018). Impact of Cigarette Smoking on the Gastrointestinal Tract Inflammation: Opposing Effects in Crohn's Disease and Ulcerative

Colitis. Frontiers in immunology, 9, 74.

32. Biedermann, L., Zeitz, J., Mwinyi, J., Sutter-Minder, E., Rehman, A., Ott, S. J., Steurer-Stey, C., Frei, A., Frei, P., Scharl, M., Loessner, M. J., Vavricka, S. R., Fried, M., Schreiber, S., Schuppler, M., & Rogler, G. (2013). Smoking cessation induces profound changes in the composition of the intestinal microbiota in humans. PloS one, 8(3), e59260.

33. Konturek, P. C., Brzozowski, T., & Konturek, S. J. (2011). Stress and the gut: pathophysiology, clinical consequences, diagnostic approach and treatment options. Journal of physiology and pharmacology : an official journal of the Polish Physiological Society, 62(6), 591–599.

34. Coquoz, A., Regli, D., & Stute, P. (2022). Impact of progesterone on the gastrointestinal tract: a comprehensive literature review. Climacteric : the journal of the International Menopause Society, 25(4), 337–361.

35. Baker, J. M., Al-Nakkash, L., & Herbst-Kralovetz, M. M. (2017). Estrogen-gut microbiome axis: Physiological and clinical implications. Maturitas, 103, 45–53.

36. Wang, J., Liu, T., Liu, L., Chen, X., Zhang, X., Du, H., Wang, C., Li, J., & Li, J. (2022). Immune dysfunction induced by 2,6-dichloro-1,4-benzoquinone, an emerging water disinfection byproduct, due to the defects of host-microbiome interactions. Chemosphere, 294, 133777.

37. Kirstein, I. V., Hensel, F., Gomiero, A., Iordachescu, L., Vianello, A., Wittgren, H. B., & Vollertsen, J. (2021). Drinking plastics? - Quantification and qualification of microplastics in drinking water distribution systems by µFTIR and Py-GCMS. Water research, 188, 116519

38. Khan, M. N., Khan, S. I., Rana, M. I., Ayyaz, A., Khan, M. Y., & Imran, M. (2022). Intermittent fasting positively modulates human gut microbial diversity and ameliorates blood lipid profile. Frontiers in microbiology, 13, 922727.

39. Pérez-Gerdel, T., Camargo, M., Alvarado, M., & Ramírez, J. D. (2023). Impact of Intermittent Fasting on the Gut Microbiota: A Systematic Review. Advanced biology, 7(8), e2200337.

Chapter 2:

1. Yang, J., Wang, H. P., Zhou, L., & Xu, C. F. (2012). Effect of dietary fiber on constipation: a meta analysis. World journal of gastroenterology, 18(48), 7378–7383.

2. Ho, K. S., Tan, C. Y., Mohd Daud, M. A., & Seow-Choen, F. (2012). Stopping or reducing dietary fiber intake reduces constipation and its associated symptoms. World Journal of Gastroenterology, 18(33), 4593-4596.

3. Peery, A. F., Sandler, R. S., Ahnen, D. J., Galanko, J. A., Holm, A. N., Shaukat, A., Mott, L. A., Barry, E. L., Fried, D. A., & Baron, J. A. (2013). Constipation and a low-fiber diet are not associated with diverticulosis. Clinical gastroenterology and hepatology : the official clinical practice journal of the American Gastroenterological Association, 11(12), 1622–1627.

4. Peery, A. F., Barrett, P. R., Park, D., Rogers, A. J., Galanko, J. A., Martin, C. F., & Sandler, R. S. (2012). A high-fiber diet does not protect against asymptomatic diverticulosis. Gastroenterology, 142(2), 266–72.e1.

5. Torre, M., Rodriguez, A. R., & Saura-Calixto, F. (1991). Effects of dietary fiber and phytic acid on mineral availability. Critical reviews in food science and nutrition, 30(1), 1–22.

6. Ames, B. N., Profet, M., & Gold, L. S. (1990). Dietary pesticides (99.99% all natural). Proceedings of the National Academy of Sciences of the United States of America, 87(19), 7777–7781.

7. Bsc, S. N., & Bsc, G. S. (1999). Oxalate content of foods and its effect on humans. Asia Pacific Journal of Clinical Nutrition, 8(1), 64-74.

8. Peck, A. B., Canales, B. K., & Nguyen, C. Q. (2016). Oxalate-degrading microorganisms or oxalate-degrading enzymes: which is the future therapy for enzymatic dissolution of calcium-oxalate uroliths in recurrent stone disease? Urolithiasis, 44(1), 45-50.

9. Frishberg, Y., Feinstein, S., Rinat, C., & Drukker, A. (2000). Hypothyroidism in primary hyperoxaluria type 1. The Journal of pediatrics, 136(2), 255–257.

10. Vojdani, A. (2015). Lectins, agglutinins, and their roles in autoimmune reactivities. Alternative Therapies in Health and Medicine, 21(Suppl 1), 46-51.

11. Ceri, H., Falkenberg-Anderson, K., Fang, R. X., Costerton, J. W., Howard, B., & Banwell, J. G. (1988). Bacteria-lectin interactions in phytohemagglutinin-induced bacterial overgrowth of the small intestine. Canadian journal of microbiology, 34(8), 1003–1008.

12. Pramod, S. N., Venkatesh, Y. P., & Mahesh, P. A. (2007). Potato lectin activates basophils and mast cells of atopic subjects by its interaction with core chitobiose of cell-bound non-specific immunoglobulin E. Clinical and experimental immunology, 148(3),

391–401.

13. Burgos-Morón, E., Calderón-Montaño, J. M., Salvador, J., Robles, A., & López-Lázaro, M. (2010). The dark side of curcumin. International journal of cancer, 126(7), 1771–1775.

14. Fang, J., Lu, J., & Holmgren, A. (2005). Thioredoxin reductase is irreversibly modified by curcumin: a novel molecular mechanism for its anticancer activity. The Journal of biological chemistry, 280(26), 25284–25290.

15. Messina M. (2016). Soy and Health Update: Evaluation of the Clinical and Epidemiologic Literature. Nutrients, 8(12), 754.

16. Bar-El, D. S., & Reifen, R. (2010). Soy as an endocrine disruptor: cause for caution?. Journal of pediatric endocrinology & metabolism : JPEM, 23(9), 855–861.

17. Habito, R. C., Montalto, J., Leslie, E., & Ball, M. J. (2000). Effects of replacing meat with soyabean in the diet on sex hormone concentrations in healthy adult males. The British journal of nutrition, 84(4), 557–563.

18. Dinsdale, E. C., & Ward, W. E. (2010). Early exposure to soy isoflavones and effects on reproductive health: a review of human and animal studies. Nutrients, 2(11), 1156–1187.

19. Jameel, F., Phang, M., Wood, L. G., & Garg, M. L. (2014). Acute effects of feeding fructose, glucose and sucrose on blood lipid levels and systemic inflammation. Lipids in Health and Disease, 13(1), 195.

20. Barnett, J. A., Bandy, M. L., & Gibson, D. L. (2022). Is the Use of Glyphosate in Modern Agriculture Resulting in Increased Neuropsychiatric Conditions Through Modulation of the Gut-brain-microbiome Axis?. Frontiers in nutrition, 9, 827384.

21. Ospina, M., Schütze, A., Morales-Agudelo, P., Vidal, M., Wong, L. Y., & Calafat, A. M. (2022). Exposure to glyphosate in the United States: Data from the 2013-2014 National Health and Nutrition Examination Survey. Environment international, 170, 107620.

Chapter 3:

1. Sauberlich, H. E. (1985). Bioavailability of vitamins. Progress in Food & Nutrition Science, 9(1-2), 1-33.

2. Haskell, M. J. (2012). The challenge to reach nutritional adequacy for vitamin A: β-carotene bioavailability and conversion—evidence in humans. The American Journal of Clinical Nutrition, 96(5), 1193S-1203S.

3. Yang, L., Zhang, Y., Wang, J., Huang, Z., Gou, L., Wang, Z., ... & Yang, X. (2016). Non-Heme Iron absorption and utilization from

typical whole Chinese diets in young Chinese urban men measured by a double-labeled stable isotope technique. PLoS One, 11(4), e0153885.

4. Daley, C. A., Abbott, A., Doyle, P. S., Nader, G. A., & Larson, S. (2010). A review of fatty acid profiles and antioxidant content in grass-fed and grain-fed beef. Nutrition journal, 9(1), 10.

5. Tang, G. (2010). Bioconversion of dietary provitamin A carotenoids to vitamin A in humans. The American Journal of Clinical Nutrition, 91(5), 1468S–1473S.

6. Trang, H. M., et al. (1998). Evidence that vitamin D3 increases serum 25-hydroxyvitamin D more efficiently than does vitamin D2. The American Journal of Clinical Nutrition, 68(4), 854-8.

7. Outila, T. A., et al. (2000). Dietary intake of vitamin D in premenopausal, healthy vegans was insufficient to maintain concentrations of serum 25-hydroxyvitamin D and intact parathyroid hormone within normal ranges during the winter in Finland. Journal of the American Dietetic Association, 100(4), 434-41.

8. Beulens, J. W., et al. (2013). The role of menaquinones (vitamin K2) in human health. British Journal of Nutrition, 110(8), 1357-68.

9. Reynolds, R. D. (1988). Bioavailability of vitamin B-6 from plant foods. The American Journal of Clinical Nutrition, 48(3 Suppl), 863-7.

10. Hooda, J., et al. (2014). Heme, an essential nutrient from dietary proteins, critically impacts diverse physiological and pathological processes. Nutrients, 6(3), 1080-1102.

11. Pawlak, R., Berger, J., & Hines, I. (2016). Iron Status of Vegetarian Adults: A Review of Literature. American Journal of Lifestyle Medicine, 12(6), 486-498.

12. Gupta, R. K., Gangoliya, S. S., & Singh, N. K. (2015). Reduction of phytic acid and enhancement of bioavailable micronutrients in food grains. Journal of Food Science and Technology, 52(2), 676-684.

13. Davis, B. C., & Kris-Etherton, P. M. (2003). Achieving optimal essential fatty acid status in vegetarians: current knowledge and practical implications. The American Journal of Clinical Nutrition, 78(3 Suppl), 640S-646S.

14. van Vliet, S., Burd, N. A., & van Loon, L. J. (2015). The Skeletal Muscle Anabolic Response to Plant- versus Animal-Based Protein Consumption. The Journal of nutrition, 145(9), 1981–1991.

15. Hertzler, S. R., Lieblein-Boff, J. C., Weiler, M., & Allgeier, C. (2020). Plant Proteins: Assessing Their Nutritional Quality and Effects on Health and Physical Function. Nutrients, 12(12), 3704.

Chapter 4:

1. Yorns, W. R., Jr, & Hardison, H. H. (2013). Mitochondrial dysfunction in migraine. Seminars in pediatric neurology, 20(3), 188–193.
2. Leeuwenburgh, C., & Heinecke, J. W. (2001). Oxidative stress and antioxidants in exercise. Current medicinal chemistry, 8(7), 829–838.

Chapter 5:

1. Gibson, A. A., Seimon, R. V., Lee, C. M., Ayre, J., Franklin, J., Markovic, T. P., Caterson, I. D., & Sainsbury, A. (2015). Do ketogenic diets really suppress appetite? A systematic review and meta-analysis. Obesity reviews : an official journal of the International Association for the Study of Obesity, 16(1), 64–76.
2. Lennerz, B. S., Mey, J. T., Henn, O. H., & Ludwig, D. S. (2021). Behavioral Characteristics and Self-Reported Health Status among 2029 Adults Consuming a "Carnivore Diet". Current developments in nutrition, 5(12), nzab133.
3. Roekenes, J., & Martins, C. (2021). Ketogenic diets and appetite regulation. Current opinion in clinical nutrition and metabolic care, 24(4), 359–363.
4. Dowis, K., & Banga, S. (2021). The Potential Health Benefits of the Ketogenic Diet: A Narrative Review. Nutrients, 13(5), 1654.
5. Pietrzak, D., Kasperek, K., Rękawek, P., & Piątkowska-Chmiel, I. (2022). The Therapeutic Role of Ketogenic Diet in Neurological Disorders. Nutrients, 14(9), 1952.
6. Cabrera-Mulero, A., Tinahones, A., Bandera, B., Moreno-Indias, I., Macías-González, M., & Tinahones, F. J. (2019). Keto microbiota: A powerful contributor to host disease recovery. Reviews in endocrine & metabolic disorders, 20(4), 415–425.
7. Ruth, M. R., Port, A. M., Shah, M., Bourland, A. C., Istfan, N. W., Nelson, K. P., Gokce, N., & Apovian, C. M. (2013). Consuming a hypocaloric high fat low carbohydrate diet for 12 weeks lowers C-reactive protein, and raises serum adiponectin and high density lipoprotein–cholesterol in obese subjects. Metabolism: clinical and experimental, 62(12), 1779–1787.
8. Hodgson, J. M., Ward, N. C., Burke, V., Beilin, L. J., & Puddey, I. B. (2007). Increased lean red meat intake does not elevate markers of oxidative stress and inflammation in humans. The Journal of nutrition, 137(2), 363–367.
9. Wang, C., Catlin, D. H., Starcevic, B., Heber, D., Ambler, C., Berman,

N., Lucas, G., Leung, A., Schramm, K., Lee, P. W., Hull, L., & Swerdloff, R. S. (2005). Low-fat high-fiber diet decreased serum and urine androgens in men. The Journal of clinical endocrinology and metabolism, 90(6), 3550–3559.

10. Volek, J. S., Sharman, M. J., Love, D. M., Avery, N. G., Gómez, A. L., Scheett, T. P., & Kraemer, W. J. (2002). Body composition and hormonal responses to a carbohydrate-restricted diet. Metabolism: clinical and experimental, 51(7), 864–870.

11. Nair, K. S., Welle, S. L., Halliday, D., & Campbell, R. G. (1988). Effect of beta-hydroxybutyrate on whole-body leucine kinetics and fractional mixed skeletal muscle protein synthesis in humans. The Journal of clinical investigation, 82(1), 198–205.

12. Vandoorne, T., De Smet, S., Ramaekers, M., Van Thienen, R., De Bock, K., Clarke, K., & Hespel, P. (2017). Intake of a Ketone Ester Drink during Recovery from Exercise Promotes mTORC1 Signaling but Not Glycogen Resynthesis in Human Muscle. Frontiers in physiology, 8, 310.

13. Volek, J. S., Freidenreich, D. J., Saenz, C., Kunces, L. J., Creighton, B. C., Bartley, J. M., Davitt, P. M., Munoz, C. X., Anderson, J. M., Maresh, C. M., Lee, E. C., Schuenke, M. D., Aerni, G., Kraemer, W. J., & Phinney, S. D. (2016). Metabolic characteristics of keto-adapted ultra-endurance runners. Metabolism: clinical and experimental, 65(3), 100–110.

14. Phinney, S. D., Bistrian, B. R., Evans, W. J., Gervino, E., & Blackburn, G. L. (1983). The human metabolic response to chronic ketosis without caloric restriction: preservation of submaximal exercise capability with reduced carbohydrate oxidation. Metabolism: clinical and experimental, 32(8), 769–776.

15. Wax, B., Kerksick, C. M., Jagim, A. R., Mayo, J. J., Lyons, B. C., & Kreider, R. B. (2021). Creatine for Exercise and Sports Performance, with Recovery Considerations for Healthy Populations. Nutrients, 13(6), 1915.

16. Dobersek, U., Teel, K., Altmeyer, S., Adkins, J., Wy, G., & Peak, J. (2023). Meat and mental health: A meta-analysis of meat consumption, depression, and anxiety. Critical reviews in food science and nutrition, 63(19), 3556–3573.

17. Ocklenburg, S., & Borawski, J. (2021). Vegetarian diet and depression scores: A meta-analysis. Journal of affective disorders, 294, 813–815.

18. LaManna, J. C., Salem, N., Puchowicz, M., Erokwu, B., Koppaka, S., Flask, C., & Lee, Z. (2009). Ketones suppress brain glucose

consumption. Advances in experimental medicine and biology, 645, 301–306.

19. Gundry, S. R. (2018). Remission/Cure of autoimmune diseases by a lectin limited diet supplemented with probiotics, prebiotics, and polyphenols. Circulation, 137

20. Peter Martin, Martina Johansson, Annelie Ek et al. A Zero Carbohydrate, Carnivore Diet can Normalize Hydrogen Positive Small Intestinal Bacterial Overgrowth Lactulose Breath Tests: A Case Report, 19 January 2021, PREPRINT (Version 1) available at Research Square

21. DiNicolantonio, J. J., & O'Keefe, J. H. (2018). The introduction of refined carbohydrates in the Alaskan Inland Inuit diet may have led to an increase in dental caries, hypertension and atherosclerosis. Journal Name, Volume(Issue), pages.

Chapter 6:

1. De Souza, R. J., Mente, A., Maroleanu, A., Cozma, A. I., Ha, V., Kishibe, T., ... & Anand, S. S. (2015). Intake of saturated and trans unsaturated fatty acids and risk of all cause mortality, cardiovascular disease, and type 2 diabetes: systematic review and meta-analysis of observational studies. BMJ, 351, h3978.

2. Malhotra, A., Redberg, R. F., & Meier, P. (2017). Saturated fat does not clog the arteries: coronary heart disease is a chronic inflammatory condition, the risk of which can be effectively reduced from healthy lifestyle interventions.

3. Dashti, H. M., Bo-Abbas, Y. Y., Asfar, S. K., Mathew, T. C., Hussein, T., Behbahani, A., ... & Al-Zaid, N. S. (2003). Ketogenic diet modifies the risk factors of heart disease in obese patients. Nutrition, 19(10), 901.

4. Brehm, B. J., Seeley, R. J., Daniels, S. R., & D'Alessio, D. A. (2003). A randomized trial comparing a very low carbohydrate diet and a calorie-restricted low fat diet on body weight and cardiovascular risk factors in healthy women. The Journal of Clinical Endocrinology & Metabolism, 88(4), 1617-1623.

5. Volek, J. S., Phinney, S. D., Forsythe, C. E., Quann, E. E., Wood, R. J., Puglisi, M. J., ... & Feinman, R. D. (2009). Carbohydrate restriction has a more favorable impact on the metabolic syndrome than a low fat diet. Lipids, 44(4), 297-309.

6. Sharman, M. J., Kraemer, W. J., Love, D. M., Avery, N. G., Gómez, A. L., Scheett, T. P., & Volek, J. S. (2002). A ketogenic diet favorably affects serum biomarkers for cardiovascular disease in normal-

weight men. The Journal of Nutrition, 132(7), 1879-1885.

7. Lee, J. E., McLerran, D. F., Rolland, B., Chen, Y., Grant, E. J., Vedanthan, R., Inoue, M., Tsugane, S., Gao, Y. T., Tsuji, I., Kakizaki, M., Ahsan, H., Ahn, Y. O., Pan, W. H., Ozasa, K., Yoo, K. Y., Sasazuki, S., Yang, G., Watanabe, T., Sugawara, Y., … Sinha, R. (2013). Meat intake and cause-specific mortality: a pooled analysis of Asian prospective cohort studies. The American journal of clinical nutrition, 98(4), 1032–1041.

8. Lindefeldt, M., Eng, A., Darban, H., Bjerkner, A., Zetterström, C. K., Allander, T., Andersson, B., Borenstein, E., Dahlin, M., & Prast-Nielsen, S. (2019). The ketogenic diet influences taxonomic and functional composition of the gut microbiota in children with severe epilepsy. NPJ biofilms and microbiomes, 5(1), 5.

9. Bui, T. P. N., Ritari, J., Boeren, S., De Waard, P., Plugge, C. M., & De Vos, W. M. (2015). Production of butyrate from lysine and the Amadori product fructoselysine by a human gut commensal. Nature Communications, 6, 10062.

10. Gu, X., Drouin-Chartier, J. P., Sacks, F. M., Hu, F. B., Rosner, B., & Willett, W. C. (2023). Red meat intake and risk of type 2 diabetes in a prospective cohort study of United States females and males. The American journal of clinical nutrition, 118(6), 1153–1163.

11. https://unsettledscience.substack.com/p/harvard-has-been-anti-meat-for-30

12. Sanders, L.M., Wilcox, M.L. & Maki, K.C. Red meat consumption and risk factors for type 2 diabetes: a systematic review and meta-analysis of randomized controlled trials. Eur J Clin Nutr 77, 156–165 (2023).

13. Bouvard, V., Loomis, D., Guyton, K. Z., Grosse, Y., Ghissassi, F. E., Benbrahim-Tallaa, L., Guha, N., Mattock, H., Straif, K., & International Agency for Research on Cancer Monograph Working Group (2015). Carcinogenicity of consumption of red and processed meat. The Lancet. Oncology, 16(16), 1599–1600.

14. Bernardi, M., & De Morais, H. A. (2019). Dietary protein intake and renal function. American Journal of Kidney Diseases, 73(3), 353-358.

15. Devries, M. C., Sithamparapillai, A., Brimble, K. S., Banfield, L., Morton, R. W., & Phillips, S. M. (2018). Changes in Kidney Function Do Not Differ between Healthy Adults Consuming Higher- Compared with Lower- or Normal-Protein Diets: A Systematic Review and Meta-Analysis. The Journal of nutrition, 148(11), 1760–1775.

16. Lieb, C. W. (1926). The effects of an exclusive, long-continued meat diet: based on the history, experiences and clinical survey of Vilhjalmur Stefansson, arctic explorer. JAMA, 87(1), 25-26.
17. Pelletier, N., Pirog, R., & Rasmussen, R. (2010). Comparative life cycle environmental impacts of three beef production strategies in the Upper Midwestern United States. Agricultural Systems, 103(6), 380-389.
18. Wolf, B., Zheng, X., Brüggemann, N., Chen, W., Dannenmann, M., Han, X., ... & Butterbach-Bahl, K. (2010). Grazing-induced reduction of natural nitrous oxide release from continental steppe. Nature, 464(7290), 881.
19. https://www.cancer.gov/about-cancer/causes-prevention/risk/diet/cooked-meats-fact-sheet
20. Kaefer, C. M., & Milner, J. A. (2008). The role of herbs and spices in cancer prevention. The Journal of nutritional biochemistry, 19(6), 347-361.
21. https://www.naturalmedicinejournal.com/journal/marinades-reduce-heterocyclic-amines-primitive-food-preparation-techniques

Chapter 7:

1. Tabatabaeizadeh, S. A., et al. (2018). Vitamin D, the gut microbiome and inflammatory bowel disease. Journal of Research in Medical Sciences, 23, 75.
2. Duggan, C., et al. (2002). Protective nutrients and functional foods for the gastrointestinal tract. The American Journal of Clinical Nutrition, 75(5), 789-808.
3. Ohashi, W., & Fukada, T. (2019). Contribution of zinc and zinc transporters in the pathogenesis of inflammatory bowel diseases. Journal of Immunology Research, 2019, Article ID 8396878.
4. Gundry, S. R. (2018). Remission/Cure of autoimmune diseases by a lectin limited diet supplemented with probiotics, prebiotics, and polyphenols. Circulation, 137

Chapter 8:

- N/A

Printed in Great Britain
by Amazon

41622067R00088